Protocols for Cardiac MR and CT

Guillem Pons-Lladó
Editor

Protocols for Cardiac MR and CT

A Guide to Study Planning and Image Interpretation

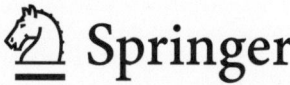 Springer

Editor
Guillem Pons-Lladó
Hospital de la Santa Creu i Sant Pau
Cardiac Imaging Unit
Cardiac Department
Barcelona
Spain

ISBN 978-3-319-30830-2   ISBN 978-3-319-30831-9 (eBook)
DOI 10.1007/978-3-319-30831-9

Library of Congress Control Number: 2016939941

© Springer International Publishing Switzerland 2016
This work is subject to copyright. All rights are reserved by the Publisher, whether the whole or part of the material is concerned, specifically the rights of translation, reprinting, reuse of illustrations, recitation, broadcasting, reproduction on microfilms or in any other physical way, and transmission or information storage and retrieval, electronic adaptation, computer software, or by similar or dissimilar methodology now known or hereafter developed.
The use of general descriptive names, registered names, trademarks, service marks, etc. in this publication does not imply, even in the absence of a specific statement, that such names are exempt from the relevant protective laws and regulations and therefore free for general use.
The publisher, the authors and the editors are safe to assume that the advice and information in this book are believed to be true and accurate at the date of publication. Neither the publisher nor the authors or the editors give a warranty, express or implied, with respect to the material contained herein or for any errors or omissions that may have been made.

Printed on acid-free paper

This Springer imprint is published by Springer Nature
The registered company is Springer International Publishing AG Switzerland

Preface

The techniques of Cardiovascular Magnetic Resonance (CMR) and Cardiac Computed Tomography (CCT) have been introduced to the diagnostic field of cardiology over the last decades, but their application is not yet fully developed in daily practice, even at large academic centres. For this reason, groups with experience in these areas are rarer than those in, say, echocardiography; thus, cardiologists and radiologists wishing to get started face the issue of finding accessible, well-oriented educational sources.

Our group began to study patients regularly with CMR in the early 1990s and CCT in the early 2000s. Both techniques, together with echocardiography, nowadays constitute the triple basis of our cardiac imaging unit, which permits a full, rational integration of these non-invasive imaging techniques into the clinical workup of cardiac patients.

This broad experience and the practical perspective acquired with our comprehensive approach led us to consider educational activities as a real commitment of our group. Thus, over recent years, several training programmes at different levels have been started, such as the Master's Degree on Advanced Imaging Techniques (CMR and CCT) endorsed by the Autonomous University of Barcelona, a 9-month, annual academic course now in its fifth edition, addressed to graduated cardiology and radiology specialists.

This handbook is the international version of a previous Spanish edition, which was first conceived as additional material for the students on the master's course to complement their practical sessions. It contained the information required to guide them through the process of acquiring, analysing and reporting CMR and CCT studies.

With this practical approach in mind, the book addresses the reader directly to the basic study protocols to apply in particular pathological processes, which are didactically described. Also, tips for the analysis of images are provided, including specific valuable data for interpreting the studies. In addition, as different imaging techniques are available in clinical practice, a rationale must be applied to choose between them. To help with this, we repeatedly discuss the uses of each technique in the diagnostic process of specific cardiovascular diseases, highlighting those aspects in which CMR and CCT are truly unique modalities in comparison with other diagnostic methods. Bibliographical references at the end of each chapter will help readers wishing to go deeper into particular issues.

We are in debt, first of all, to our students for their stimulus to write this book, to which all of them have directly, or indirectly, contributed with their comments and questions when attending the practical sessions. Clinical users of these techniques, particularly non-radiologists, usually have limited authority in physics or in the technical aspects of MR and CT systems, and this is why we asked Mr. Javier Sánchez, Clinical Scientist at Philips Ibérica, for his support in these issues. This does not mean, however, that the book is restricted to users of this company, as the cardiac MR sequences and cardio CT strategies described are also applicable to other equivalent systems.

For a programme of CMR and CCT to be successful in practice, a truly collaborative effort of cardiologists and radiologists is essential. This integrated approach has been possible in our centre, thanks to the chairmen of the cardiology and radiology departments, Professors Juan Cinca and Antoni Capdevila, respectively, whose personal, positive attitudes must also be acknowledged with gratitude.

We hope readers of this book take real advantage of what it provides, which is a concise but comprehensive compendium of the experience of our group in CMR and CCT that may be useful for others to start their own.

Barcelona, Spain   Guillem Pons-Lladó

Contents

1. **Magnetic Resonance Sequences for Cardiovascular Applications and Study Planning** 1
   Guillem Pons-Lladó, Alberto Hidalgo, and Sandra Pujadas

2. **CMR Study Protocol of Ischemic Heart Disease** 33
   Sandra Pujadas and Guillem Pons-Lladó

3. **CMR Study Protocol of Cardiomyopathies** 49
   Sandra Pujadas and Guillem Pons-Lladó

4. **CMR Study Protocol of Pericardial Diseases** 71
   Francesc Carreras

5. **CMR Study Protocol of Cardiac Masses and Tumours** 81
   Francesc Carreras and Alberto Hidalgo

6. **CMR Study Protocol for Great Vessels** 93
   Guillem Pons-Lladó

7. **CMR Study Protocol for Valvular Diseases** 101
   Francesc Carreras and Guillem Pons-Lladó

8. **CMR Study Protocols for Congenital Heart Diseases** 115
   Alberto Hidalgo

9. **Protocols for Cardiac Studies with Computed Tomography** 131
   Rubén Leta and Antonio Barros

10. **Cardiac Computed Tomography: Post-processing and Analysis** 143
    Rubén Leta and Antonio Barros

Magnetic Resonance Sequences for Cardiovascular Applications and Study Planning

Guillem Pons-Lladó, Alberto Hidalgo, and Sandra Pujadas

1.1 The Concept of Pulse Sequences

The correct planning of cardiovascular magnetic resonance (CMR) studies requires basic knowledge of both the various types of pulse sequences with applications in cardiology and of the heart's anatomy. Using this knowledge we can obtain images with adequate tissue contrast and the anatomical orientation necessary for their analysis.

The sequences of acquisition of MR images are computer programmes (software) that organise the application of radiofrequency pulses and magnetic field gradients into a chronogram to modulate the characteristics of the signal received and with it the appearance of the resulting image. The different sequences exercise precise control over the basic elements of the functioning of the MR systems (hardware) such as the emission of pulses by the radiofrequency transmitters that interact with the atomic nuclei to produce the phenomenon of magnetic resonance and generate linear magnetic field gradients which allow special codification of the signal received.

As a result of the application of the MR sequences, it is possible to modulate the intensity of the signal received in such a way that certain specific magnetic properties of the tissues can be highlighted, such as the magnetisation recovery time (T1) and the signal degradation after an excitation (T2), which gives MR its capacity to analyse different tissue characteristics. The use of paramagnetic contrast is another of the technique's resources. Using contrast the vascularisation of the tissues or the state of the perfusion can be assessed based on the changes in the magnetic properties of the tissues after the contrast agent reaches the tissue's microvascular network.

G. Pons-Lladó, MD, PhD (✉) • S. Pujadas, MD
Cardiac Imaging Unit, Cardiology Department, Hospital de la Santa Creu i Sant Pau,
Universitat Autònoma de Barcelona, Barcelona, Spain
e-mail: gpons@santpau.cat

A. Hidalgo, MD, PhD
Cardiac Imaging Unit, Radiology Department, Hospital de la Santa Creu i Sant Pau,
Universitat Autònoma de Barcelona, Barcelona, Spain

1.2 The Basis of Sequence Acquisition in CMR

Generally, CMR images are acquired in slices or two-dimensional (2D) sections 5–10 mm thick, with an in-plane resolution of between 1 and 2 mm. The acquisition is synchronised with the cardiac cycle using an electrocardiogram (ECG) or peripheral pulse signal as a reference, making it possible to divide the cardiac cycle into different segments of time. For adequate temporal representation of the heart's movement during a cardiac cycle, it is necessary to segment the cycle into time windows of the order of 20 ms (30 phases per cardiac cycle). Within this narrow time frame, the system cannot acquire all the information required to generate a whole image with adequate temporal resolution. To overcome this limitation, advantage is taken of the cyclical nature of the heart's movement, and the acquisition of all the information contained in the final image is extracted over several beats, generating an image with the adequate spatial and temporal resolution. This whole process is usually carried out while the patient is holding their breath (breath hold, apnoea), as respiratory movements can introduce a positional artefact to the image of the heart. Sequences that use EchoNavigator synchronisation provide an alternative to apnoea. Here, the system monitors the respiratory cycle based on the displacement of the diaphragm and only considers information gathered in phases with a specific diaphragm position.

1.3 Types of Sequences with Applications in CMR

A detailed discussion of the physical bases of MR and of the structure of the sequences is not the aim of this work, and for these purposes the recommended bibliography may be consulted. It is, however, important to have precise knowledge of the type of information the various sequences provide and to be aware of their applications in cardiovascular studies. The profusion of available sequences and their continual evolution has generated a degree of confusion, exacerbated by the various manufacturers of MR systems giving different names to otherwise equivalent sequences. Below, we describe the sequences of application for cardiac studies along with their main modification strategies. Although the names of the sequences correspond to those from one particular company (Philips), they can be found under equivalent names from other vendors.

- Black-blood *turbo spin echo (BB-TSE)*: generically called "black blood", as the signal from the moving blood flow is suppressed before the acquisition of the anatomical information and appears black. The acquisition of "black-blood" sequences may be weighted towards either T1 or T2. In both cases, a single image is obtained at a unique temporal position in the cardiac cycle. Their excellent resolution and contrast make these sequences useful for the definition of anatomical structures. Each slice is usually obtained during breath hold (see Fig. 1.1a).
- *Single-shot TSE*: a special modality of the previous sequence where every image is acquired in a single echo train providing one image per acquisition and one

acquisition per cardiac cycle, which allows multiple slices to be acquired in one breath hold, though with limited spatial resolution.
- *Short tau inversion recovery (STIR)*: a TSE sequence that is modified to suppress the signal from the adipose tissue and which is also sensitive to the presence of the tissue water component (oedema) (see Fig. 1.1b).
- *Gradient echo/fast field echo (FFE)*: the basic modality of what are generically called "bright blood" sequences due to the higher signal intensity of the blood flow compared to that from solid tissues such as the myocardium. These sequences allow a series of consecutive images to be obtained within the period of the cardiac cycle, and for this reason they are suitable for studies of cardiac function.
- *Steady-state free precession (SSFP) – (balanced FFE or balanced TFE)*: a modification of FFE/TFE sequences that allows for improved signal/noise relation; for this reason, it is currently the application of choice for functional studies (see Fig. 1.1c).
- *Echo-planar imaging (EPI)*: a mode of readout of the image information that can be applied to both spin-echo sequences and gradient echo ones, which allows shorter image acquisition time at the expense of lower resolution and/or greater sensitivity to susceptibility artefacts.
- *Turbo field echo (TFE)*: a sequence that is similar to the FFE sequences in which the generation of different phase encoding echoes are grouped into segments or trains of echoes and in which before each of those segments different prepulses may be applied.
- *Inversion recovery turbo field echo (IR-TFE)*: a modification of TFE sequences where, before each train of echoes, an inversion prepulse is applied to give greater weighting to T1 effects on the image. In delayed contrast enhancement studies, the appropriate inversion time between the prepulse and image readout must be chosen to allow signal from certain tissues, such as the healthy ventricular myocardium, to be suppressed, thus enabling the recognition of those (abnormal) regions where contrast may have been retained due to slower washout (see Fig. 1.1d).
- *Modified look locker imaging (MOLLI)*: is a special application of IR-TFE used for the estimation of actual values of T1 time in the myocardial tissue. In this sequence the same inversion pulse is shared between different heart cycles and combined with single-shot TFE acquisition in every heartbeat to increase the inversion time range to allow accurate T1 estimation.
- *Saturation recovery turbo field echo (TFE)*: a modification of TFE sequences where, before each train of echoes, a prepulse of saturation is applied to achieve greater T1 effect on the image. In contrast to the IR sequences, the image signal is independent from the signal evolution before the saturation prepulse is applied, meaning that the signal intensity of the image is always equivalent after each saturation pulse. This fact, combined with the TFE sequence acquisition speed, allows multiple slices to be taken in a single cardiac cycle with adequate resolution to detect the increase in signal produced by the arrival of contrast, which makes it useful for studies of myocardial perfusion during the first pass of a contrast agent given as an intravenous bolus (see Fig. 1.1e).

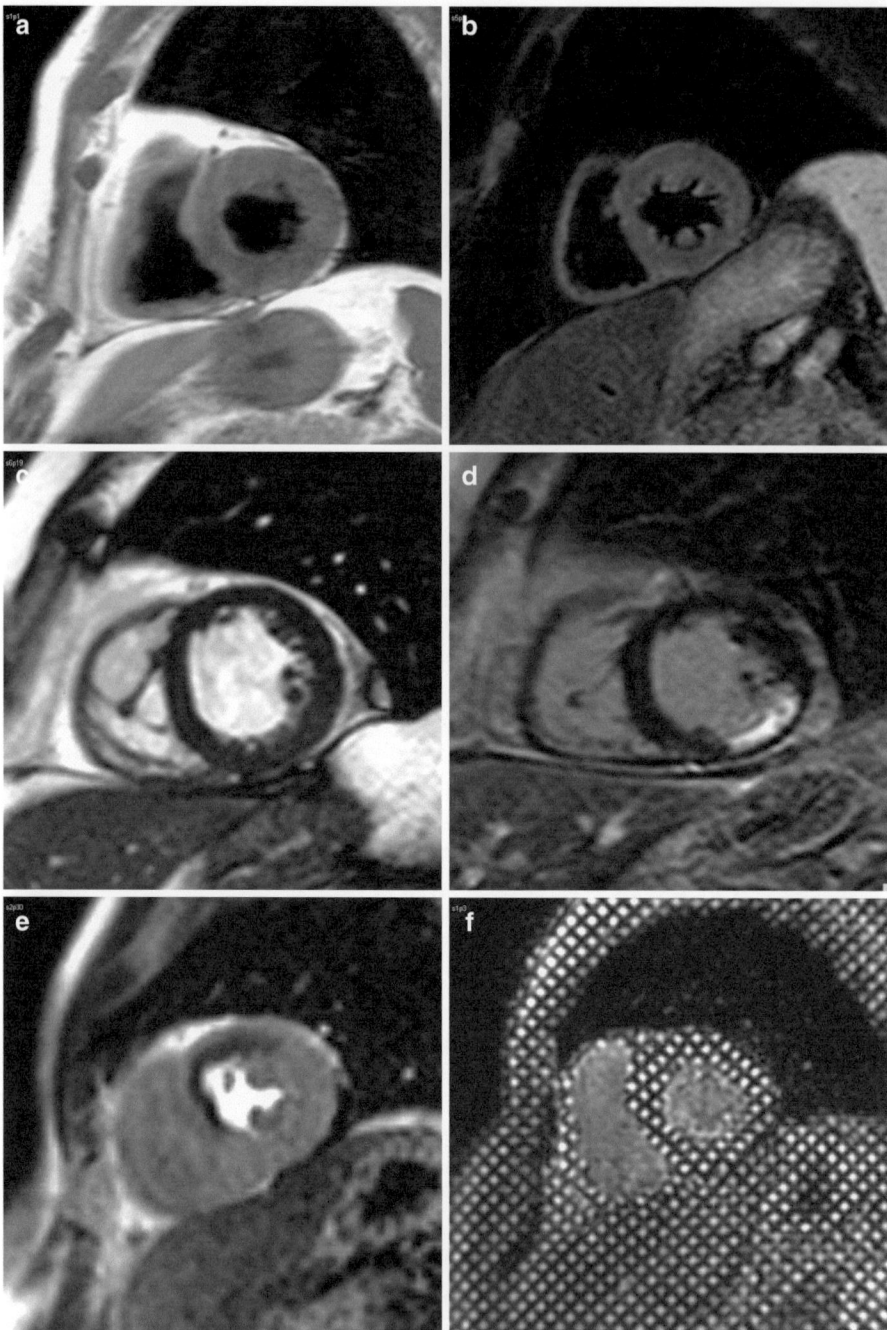

Fig 1.1 (a) Black-blood turbo spin-echo image; (b) STIR image; (c) SSFP image; (d) inversion recovery image obtained late after gadolinium contrast injection showing enhancement (*bright signal*) at the inferolateral wall of the left ventricle; (e) first-pass perfusion image showing a defect (*dark signal*) at the anteroseptal wall; (f) tagging image; (g) phase contrast image; (h) MR contrast angiography image

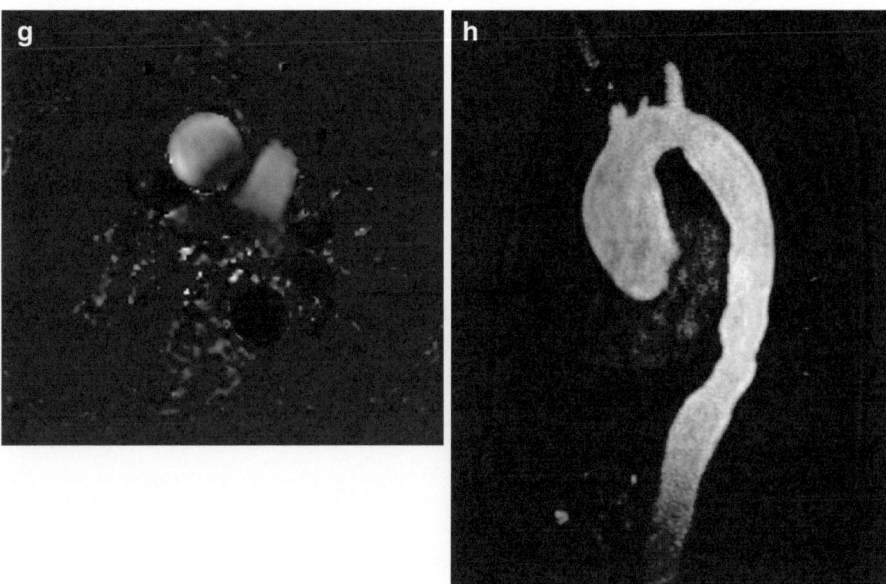

Fig 1.1 (continued)

- *Tagging*: turbo field echo or modified echo planar sequence in which, before reading an echo train, a spatial modulation of the signal intensity is applied and remains visible for a short period of time. The signal degrades over the cardiac cycle, but is still useful as a marker that allows myocardial deformation to be tracked during ventricular contraction and relaxation (see Fig. 1.1f).
- *Phase contrast (PCA)*: gradient echo or turbo gradient echo sequence modified to be able to codify flow rates by applying a magnetic field gradient within which protons in movement acquire a phase variation proportional to the flow velocity. The sequence provides instantaneous velocity curves for vascular structures with circulating blood flow (see Fig. 1.1g).
- *Whole-heart coronary MRA*: turbo SSFP sequence with T2 weighting and fat saturation acquired with respiratory navigation, which allows for multiple high-resolution slices to be taken in the same phase of the cycle with the possibility of three-dimensional (3D) reconstruction to evaluate the coronary arteries without needing to apply contrast. It is usually combined with T2 prepulses to increase contrast between the blood pool and the tissues.
- *Contrast-enhanced MR angiography*: gradient echo sequence of a 3D volume composed of multiple thin slices acquired without cardiac synchronisation during the first pass of an injection of paramagnetic contrast with the possibility of 3D reconstruction. Used for vascular angiographic studies (see Fig, 1.1h).
- *Parallel imaging technique/sensitivity encoding (SENSE)*: these are less acquisition sequences themselves than modification techniques to be combined with them. Basically, these MR imaging reconstruction techniques use the spatial

variation of the receiver coils' sensitivity as information for spatial encoding, being able thus to skip phase encoding lines during the acquisition and therefore shorten the acquisition time.

1.4 Planning and Analysis of CMR Studies

The basis of planning a CMR study is the acquisition of slices with adequate orientation relative to the axes of the heart. As the heart's position in the thorax aligns with none of the three natural anatomical planes (axial, coronal and sagittal), it is necessary to start by taking a number of images of the thorax along those standard planes in order to visualise the position of the heart and plan the study. This series of slices is called a "scout" or "localiser" and is made up of images taken in a sequence with relatively low resolution and quick acquisition, which is performed during breath hold (see Fig. 1.2).

1.4.1 Study of Heart Function

1.4.1.1 Taking Images for a Study of Function

1. The study begins by selecting an axial image from the scout series where the location of both the apex and the base of the left ventricle may be identified (see Fig. 1.2, boxed image, lower row). Based on this image, we can plan the first slice that is truly oriented along one of the heart's natural planes. The usual procedure is to use a turbo *SSFP (balanced TFE)* sequence, with a single slice of 8 mm thickness that encompasses the apex of the heart and the midpoint of the mitral valve ring (see Fig 1.3, left), from which a plane called *vertical longitudinal* or, more expressively, a two-chamber view (left atrium and ventricle) results (see Fig. 1.3, right). This sequence can be planned with the application of a method of parallel acquisition (*SENSE*), which substantially reduces the apnoea time and usually provides between 20 and 30 phases of the cardiac cycle, depending on heart rate. A cine sequence may be reconstructed in which it is possible to analyse the dynamics of the anterior and inferior regions of the left ventricle.
2. The next step consists of repeating the same sequence using the previous two-chamber view as a reference from which to take a new, orthogonal slice at the level of the approximate equatorial plane of the left ventricle (see Fig. 1.4).
3. The step described is in fact an intermediate one, as it only provides one of the required planes for obtaining the next slice, which, in contrast with the two previous ones, requires a double orientation (see Fig. 1.5): on one side, on the two-chamber plane, it is again aligned with the region of the apex and the midpoint of the mitral valve ring (see Fig. 1.5, upper right image), and, on the other side, it is aligned along the plane that runs perpendicular to this, crossing the left and right ventricles at their maximum diameters (see Fig. 1.5, lower left image). The resulting slice is called *horizontal longitudinal* or a four-chamber view (both atria and both ventricles) (see Fig. 1.5, right image).

1 Magnetic Resonance Sequences for Cardiovascular Applications and Study Planning

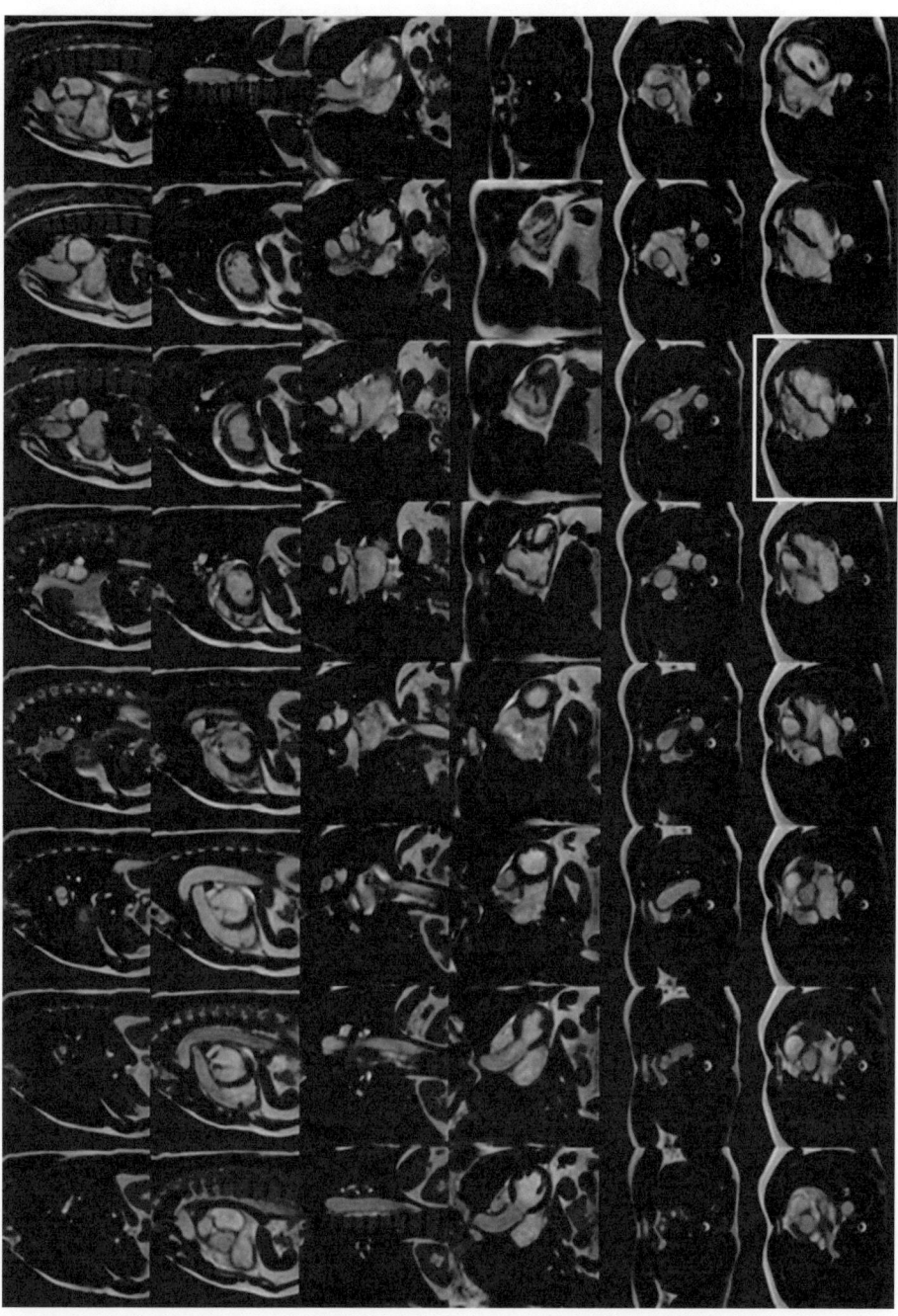

Fig. 1.2 Scout images on sagittal, coronal and transverse planes

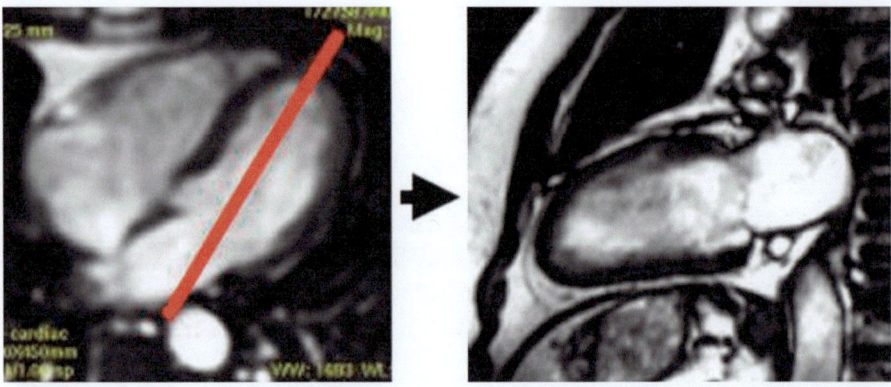

Fig. 1.3 Planning of a vertical longitudinal plane of the heart (*two*-chamber) on a scout axial slice (*left*) and the resultant image (*right*)

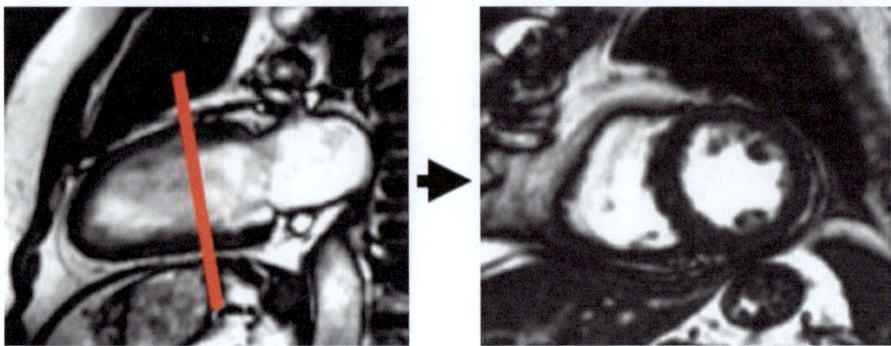

Fig. 1.4 Planning of a short-axis plane on a two-chamber slice (*left*) and the resultant image (*right*)

4. This step is optional and may be of use if a more precise two-chamber plane is required because of dissatisfaction with the first slices acquired (see Fig. 1.6). The two-chamber plane thus obtained is similar to the one described in the first step of the study, but in this case it is absolutely centred.
5. Based on the previous longitudinal planes, and using the same *turbo SSFP* sequence, a new prescription is made, this time comprising a series of parallel slices on the ventricular *short-axis* planes, covering the whole extension of both ventricles from base to apex (see Fig. 1.7). The thickness of the slices is again 8 mm. An interslice gap of 2 mm may be left, and the total number of slices is usually 10, although this will depend on the size of the ventricles. The slices should be completely parallel to the mitral and tricuspid rings; otherwise both atrial and ventricular cavities may enter the image plane and cause confusion.

1.4.1.2 Practical Aspects of Function Imaging

The use of the *SENSE* acceleration method allows the rapid acquisition of short-axis planes, making it possible to obtain several (two or three) in a single breath hold of reasonable duration.

1 Magnetic Resonance Sequences for Cardiovascular Applications and Study Planning

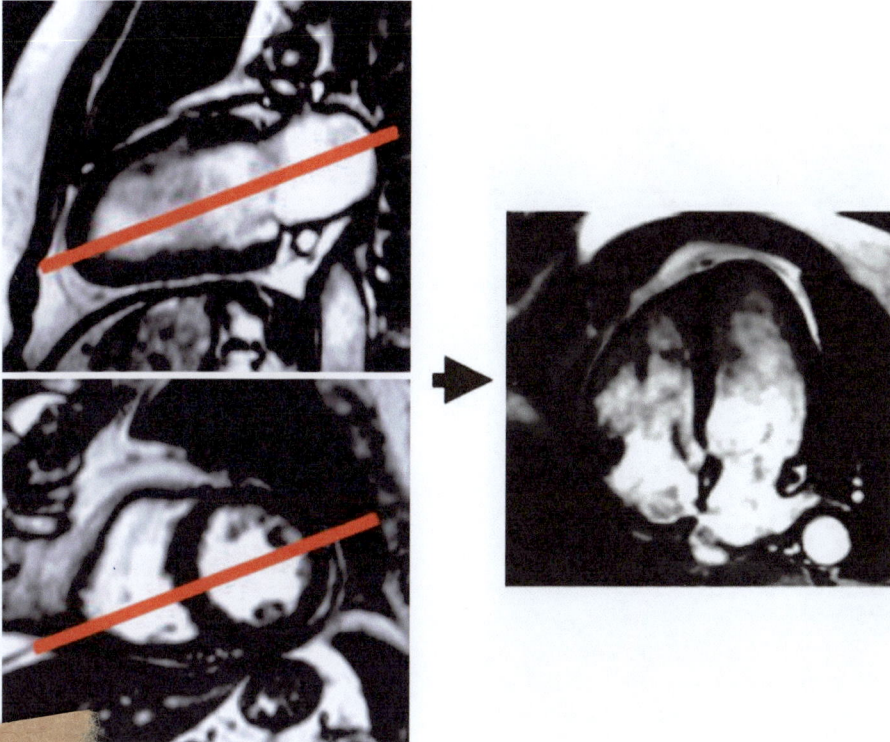

Fig. 1.5 Planning of an horizontal longitudinal plane of the heart (*four*-chamber) by double angulation on two-chamber and short-axis planes (*left*) and the resultant image (*right*)

The cine sequences described are obtained using a mode of acquisition that is retrospectively synchronised with the ECG (or pulse wave). In order to ensure adequate synchronisation of the images, the system has a mechanism of arrhythmia rejection that allows it to delete from the readout those beats that show a predetermined degree of variation in their cycle relative to the base. This means that the total times of both the acquisition and the breath hold are prolonged. In the case of very frequent premature contractions or very irregular atrial fibrillation, it may be better to switch the acquisition to a prospective method and deactivate the arrhythmia rejection to obtain a sequence that is less robust but still reasonable in duration. Another alternative is to widen the acceptance window for variations in heart rate in the arrhythmia rejection mode.

1.4.1.3 Image Analysis: Function

With the multiple short-axis cine series, we have a data set that contains information on the volume of both ventricles and the myocardial mass, as well as their changes during the phases of the cardiac cycle. The information that may be extracted from it on ventricular function and structure is, then, potentially highly valuable, but only when analysed in a careful and appropriate way.

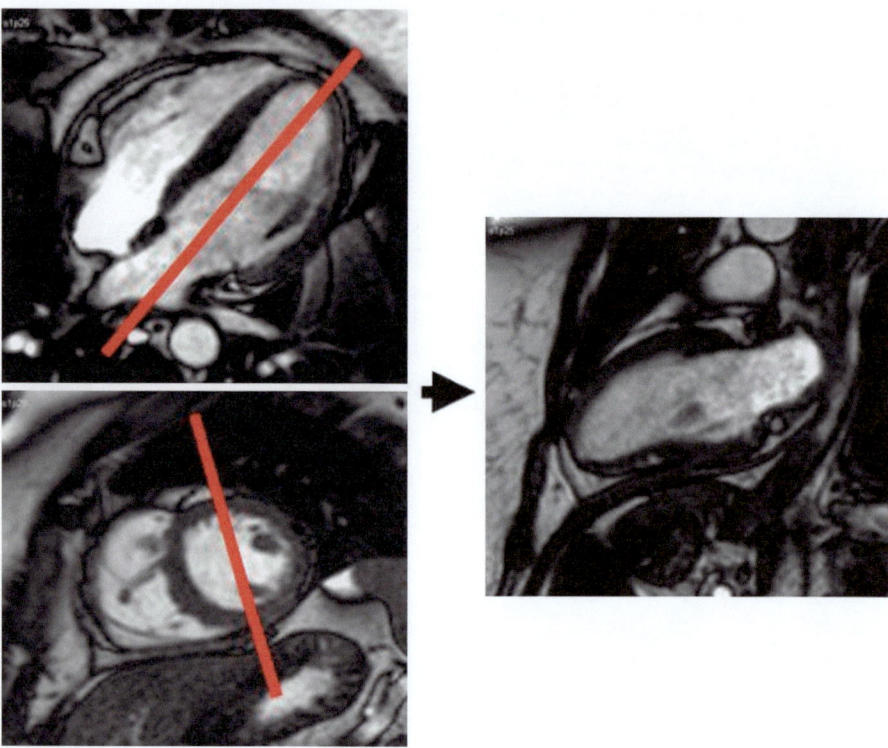

Fig. 1.6 Planning of a refined two-chamber plane by double angulation on four-chamber and short-axis planes (*left*) and the resultant image (*right*)

The images of the cine series obtained in the short axis are evaluated at a workstation. For this, the endocardial and epicardial borders of each ventricle are traced separately, either manually or automatically (which often requires subsequent manual correction) (see Fig. 1.8). The extension of this process to all the short-axis slices in all phases of the cardiac cycle provides information on the volumes and mass of both ventricles, as well as of their derived parameters, such as the ejected volume and the ejection fraction.

Analysis of regional contractile function is often made visually: segmental motion may then be considered normal, hypokinetic, akinetic or dyskinetic. However, the analysis programmes include tools to highlight such alterations through the measurement of changes in the ventricular wall thickness throughout the cardiac cycle for a particular segment (see Fig. 1.9, upper panels), showing the thickness at end-diastole and end-systole in a graph (see Fig. 1.9, lower left panel). Or, if the contours have been traced in all phases of the cardiac cycle, the segmental thickening throughout the whole cycle will be shown (see Fig. 1.9, lower right panel).

1 Magnetic Resonance Sequences for Cardiovascular Applications and Study Planning   11

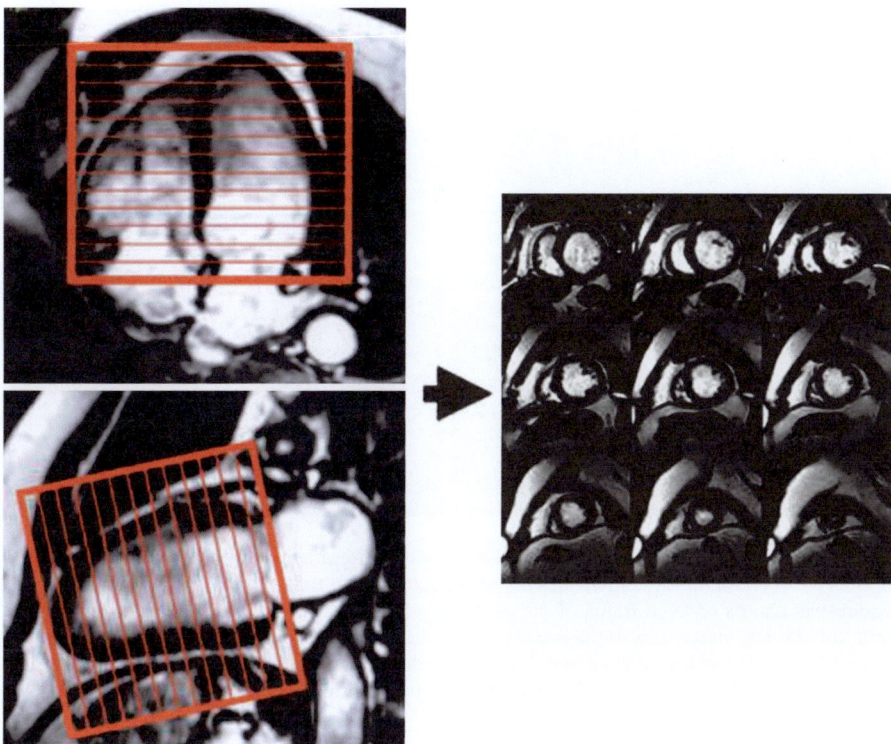

Fig. 1.7 Planning of multiple short-axis series of the ventricles on four- and two-chamber planes (*left*) and the resultant images (*right*)

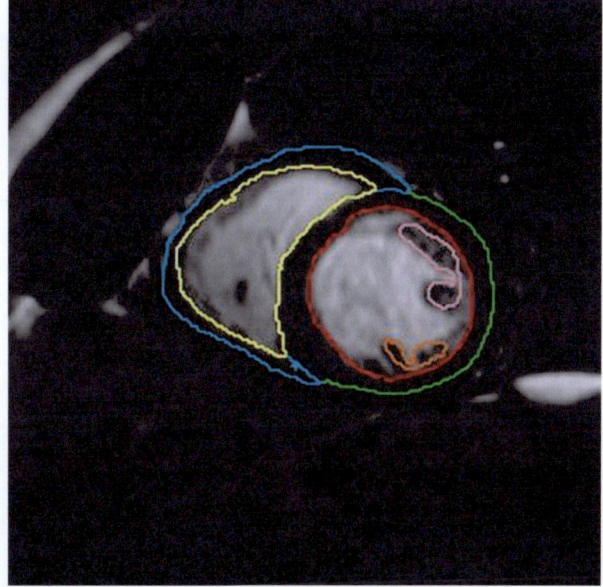

Fig. 1.8 Tracing of epicardial and endocardial contours from both ventricles and of papillary muscles for quantitation of ventricular mass and volume

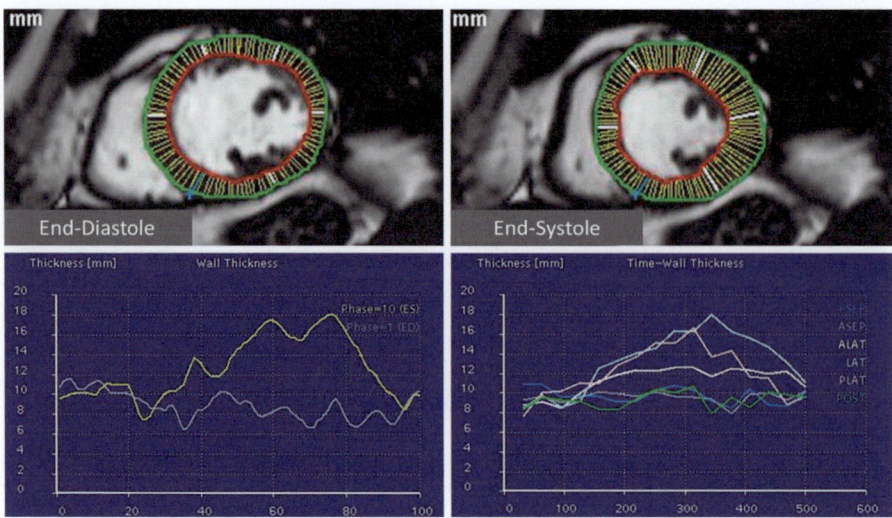

Fig. 1.9 Computer analysis of segmental wall motion. After tracing of epi- and endocardial borders by the operator, the system divides the whole extension of the left ventricle into a series of 100 equidistant chords on each frame of the cardiac cycle (*upper panels*), which can be analysed in terms of absolute values of wall thickness for each chord at end-diastole and end-systole (*lower left panel*), or as segmental wall thickening over the cardiac cycle (*lower right panel*). Segmental wall motion abnormalities are recognised by a defective increase in wall thickness at end-systole

1.4.1.4 Practical Aspects of Function Image Analysis

In order to optimise the time of the analysis, the tracing of the contours is usually performed only on those images corresponding to the end-diastolic (maximal ventricular volume) (see Fig. 1.10, left panel) and end-systolic phases (minimal ventricular volume) (see Fig. 1.10, right panel).

For the same reason, the epicardial contours of the right ventricle are often left out, as the right ventricular mass is not a commonly used parameter. Neither are the epicardial contours of the left ventricle in systole (see Fig. 1.10), given that the left ventricular mass should not vary from diastole to systole.

The papillary muscles must be included, in principle, as myocardial mass, and not as part of the ventricular volume (see Figs. 1.8 and 1.10). Nevertheless, not including them does not substantially affect the calculations of ventricular mass and volume, and they can be left out when tracing the contours in favour of greater simplicity of analysis.

Special attention should be given to the basal slices, as, owing to the longitudinal shortening of the heart in systole it may occur that, in one slice, the end-diastolic image effectively includes the ventricular cavity (see Fig. 1.11, left column), while the systolic image of the same plane corresponds to the atrium, which should not, logically, be included in the ventricular volume (see Fig. 1.11, right column). With the aim of minimising the possibility that the basal slices include, simultaneously, portions of the atrium and ventricle, it is important that the most basal one is perfectly aligned with the atrioventricular plane.

1 Magnetic Resonance Sequences for Cardiovascular Applications and Study Planning

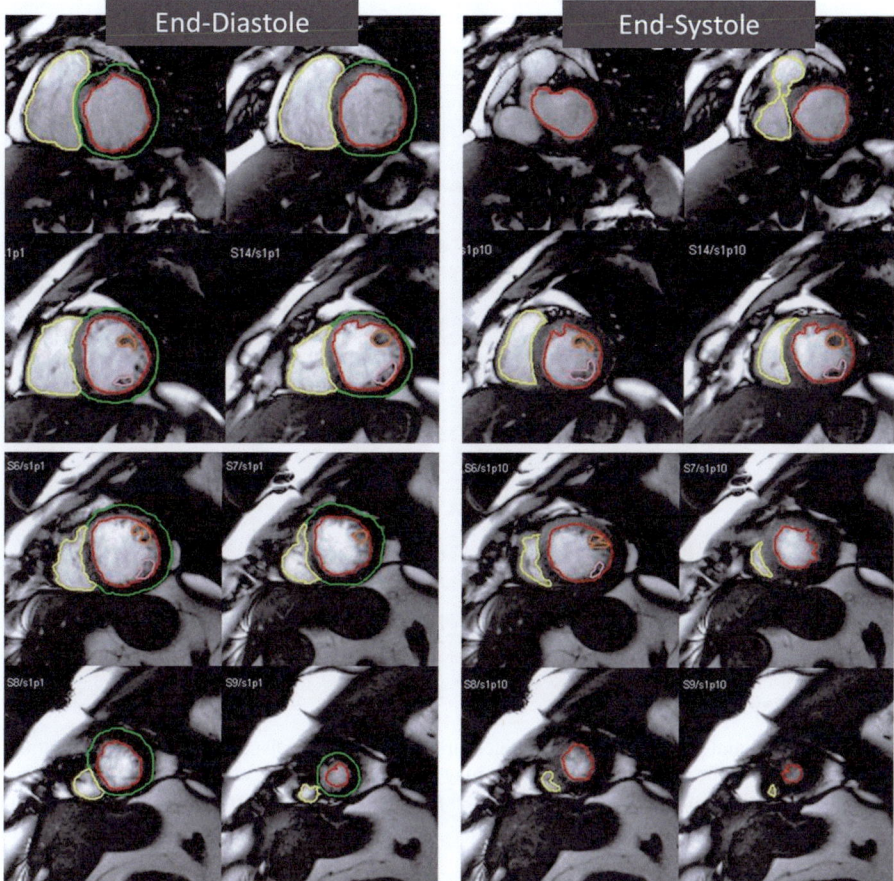

Fig. 1.10 Tracing of ventricular contours on the complete set of short-axis planes of the ventricles at both end-diastole (*left panel*) and end-systole (*right panel*)

A quick alternative to the calculation of volumes and function on short-axis planes is to apply simple area/length formulas to diastolic and systolic images on a longitudinal plane in a similar way to echocardiography (see Fig. 1.12). This calculation is acceptable as long as there are no regional alterations in contractility.

1.4.2 Cardiac Morphology Study

The cardiac function study protocol with *balanced TFE* sequences described is applied practically systematically in CMR studies and, in fact, its images provide morphological information. "Black-blood" sequences are, nevertheless, more appropriate for this purpose, as they allow each tissue's own magnetic properties to be highlighted, such as magnetisation recovery times after the emission of

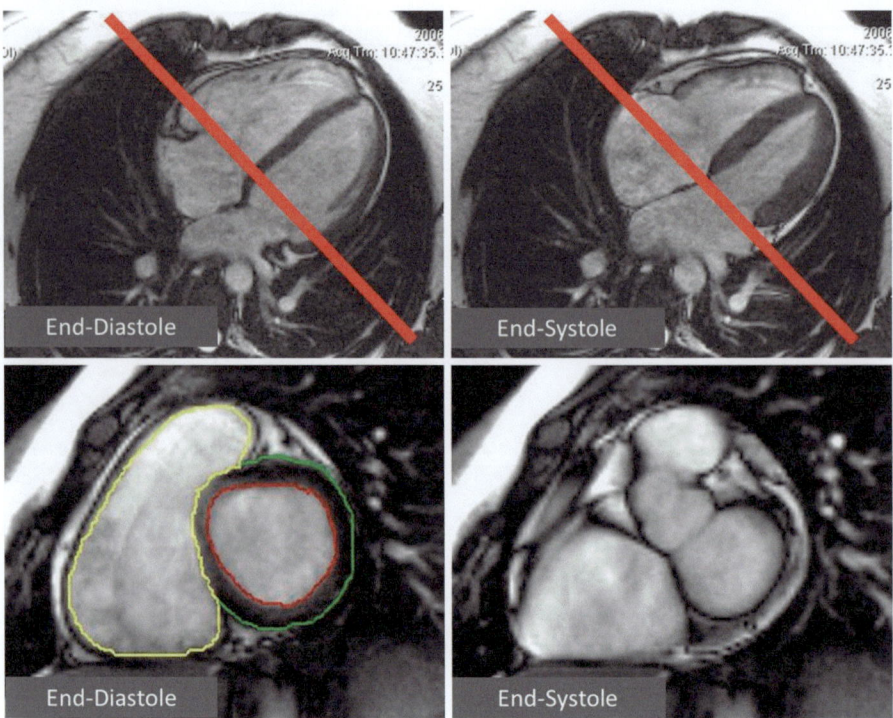

Fig. 1.11 Potential pitfall of the volume measurement due to the displacement of the base of the ventricles towards the apex in systole, which may lead to a shift in the actual contents of the imaging plane from the ventricles at end-diastole (*left panels*) to the atria at end-systole (*right panels*)

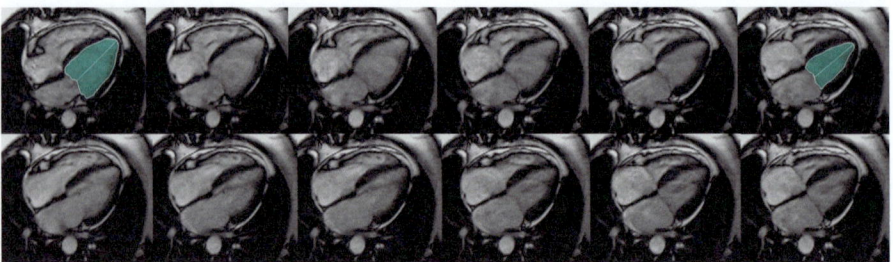

Fig. 1.12 Frames of a cine sequence on four-chamber plane where end-diastolic and end-systolic images are chosen to trace the area and length of the left ventricle for a simplified measurement of volume and function of the chamber

radiofrequency pulses (T1 and T2). In "black-blood" sequences, such T1 or T2 weighting is obtained, essentially, by modifying two parameters: repetition time (TR) and echo time of (TE). In this way, native properties of different tissues are highlighted, which allows an estimate of their nature and structure.

1.4.2.1 Acquiring Morphological Images

As this kind of sequence provides information not only on the heart but also on the paracardiac and mediastinal structures, it is usual to obtain a series of slices on a purely axial plane from the region of the pulmonary artery to the level of the inferior vena cava, with a T1-weighted *turbo spin-echo* sequence (see Fig. 1.13). This sequence provides static images in a single phase of the cardiac cycle. Using a slice thickness of 8 mm with interslice spaces of 2 mm, 10–12 slices are necessary. If high spatial resolution is required, they must be performed with one breath hold per slice.

"Black-blood" sequences weighted to T2 are appropriate for studies of myocardial characterisation, and, consequently, they are normally obtained on anatomical cardiac planes, either longitudinal or on the short axis, using a *STIR* sequence that suppresses the adipose tissue and enhances, with high signal intensity, the presence of myocardial oedema, which is a common component in a series of pathological processes of the cardiac muscle (see Fig. 1.14, arrow).

1.4.2.2 Morphological Image Analysis

The detection and quantification of the myocardial oedema are possible with the analysis of signal intensities in regions of interest (ROIs): myocardial signal that is stronger than that of the skeletal muscle by a ratio of >2 is considered indicative of myocardial oedema (see Fig. 1.15, right panel).

1.4.3 Study of Delayed Contrast Enhancement

These sequences are useful for detecting areas of myocardial tissue where the retention of contrast is abnormal due to altered distribution kinetics. This alteration may have several causes, the principal of which is the presence of a myocardial scar as a

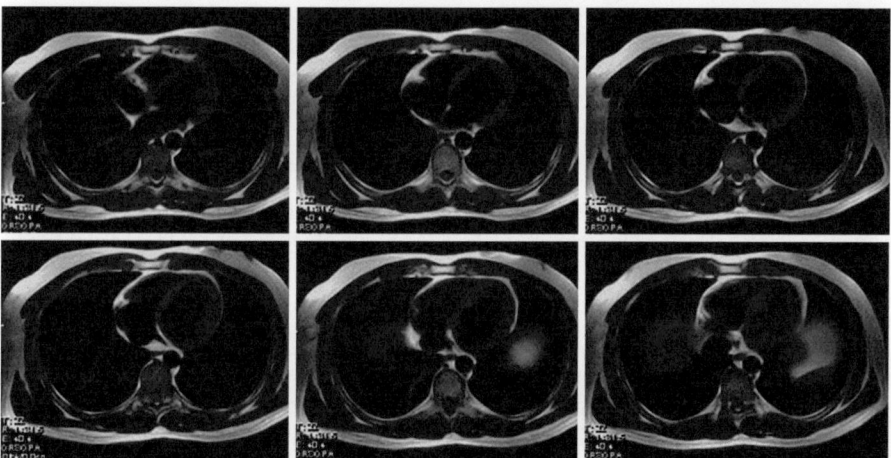

Fig. 1.13 Series of transverse planes from a black-blood turbo spin-echo sequence

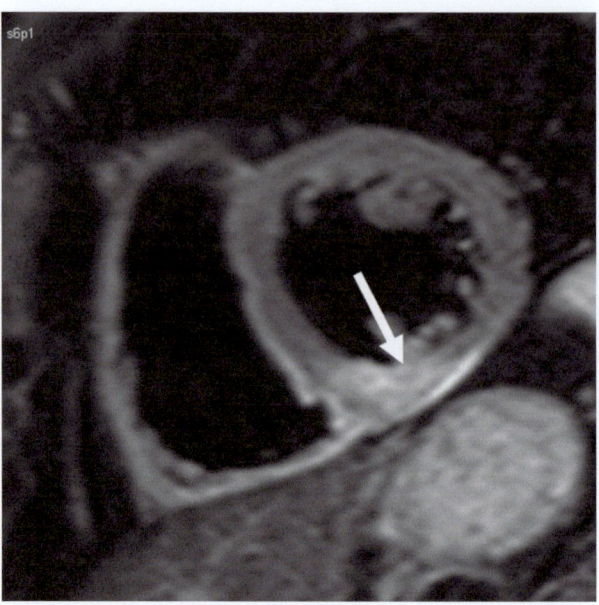

Fig. 1.14 Image from a STIR sequence showing an area of increased signal intensity (*arrow*) due to myocardial oedema

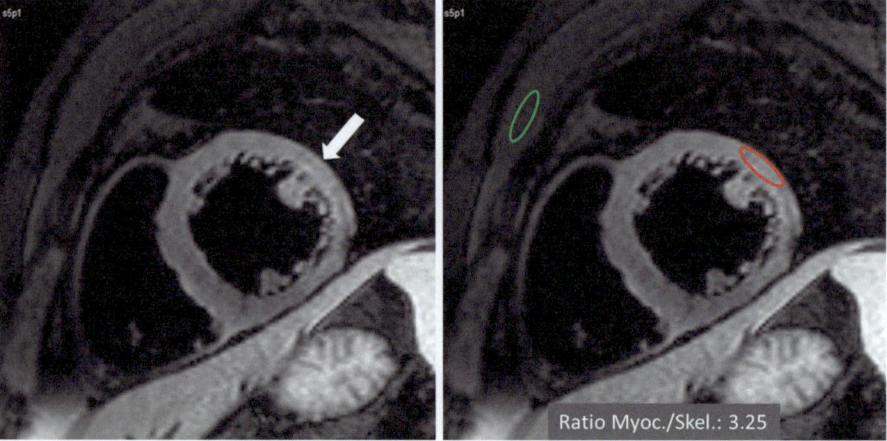

Fig. 1.15 Recognition of abnormal increase in myocardial signal intensity on STIR images (*arrow*, in the *left panel*) by the ratio of values at the region of interest and at the skeletal muscle (*right panel*)

remnant of a previous infarction. For the study of delayed contrast enhancement, an *inversion recovery turbo field echo (IR-TFE)* sequence is used which at each excitation emits a pulse of inversion of the magnetisation. The acquisition is made after the specific time (inversion time, TI) in which, during the process of magnetisation recovery, the signal in the normal myocardium is nullified, appearing thus with a low (dark) signal intensity. The presence of contrast retained in areas of damaged myocardium (by virtue of altered kinetics) is detected by an increase in signal (bright), as these areas exhibit faster magnetisation recovery than the remote myocardium.

1.4.3.1 Obtaining the Delayed Contrast Images

1. The study must be preceded by the intravenous administration of paramagnetic contrast (gadolinium), in a dose of 0.1–0.2 mmol/kg weight. The acquisition sequence begins 10 min after the injection of contrast.
2. Using the initial scout planes, or any of those obtained in previous sequences, a special sequence called *Look-Locker* is programmed, which is oriented on a short-axis ventricular plane, and consists of repeated acquisition of images, each with a progressively longer TI (see Fig. 1.16). The inspection of all the images must allow the identification of the one in which the nullification of the healthy myocardial signal is optimal (black) (see Fig. 1.16, boxed image on the upper row). The TI corresponding to this image is the one to be used for the acquisition of the subsequent IR sequence.
3. The *IR-TFE* sequence consists of a series of parallel, contiguous static slices, oriented along the longitudinal horizontal (four-chamber) and vertical (two-chamber) planes, as well as on the short axis from the ventricular base to its apex, with slice thickness and interslice gaps equal to those in the cine series and with the TI predetermined in the *Look-Locker* sequence. The presence of myocardial areas with delayed contrast enhancement is easily identified by the bright signal displayed in comparison with remote areas of non-enhanced myocardium, which show a dark signal intensity (see Fig. 1.17).

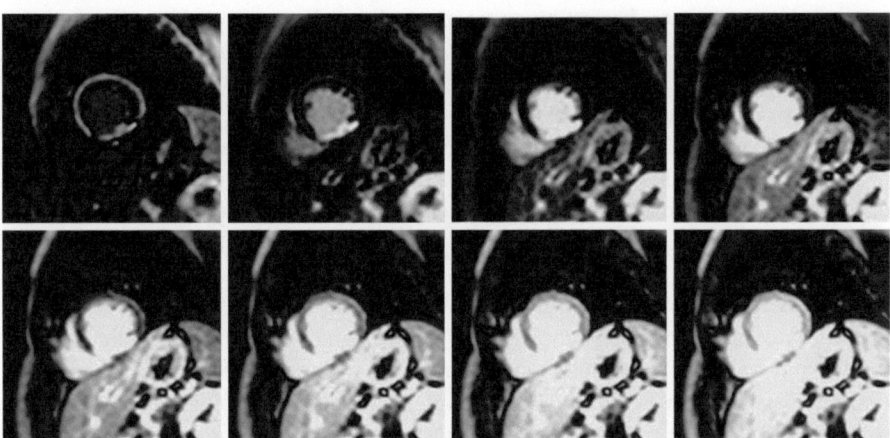

Fig. 1.16 Set of scout images with progressively longer inversion time for choosing of the appropriate one in a delayed enhancement study. The optimal value is that corresponding to the image where the signal from the left ventricular (healthy) myocardium is mostly suppressed (third frame from the *upper row*)

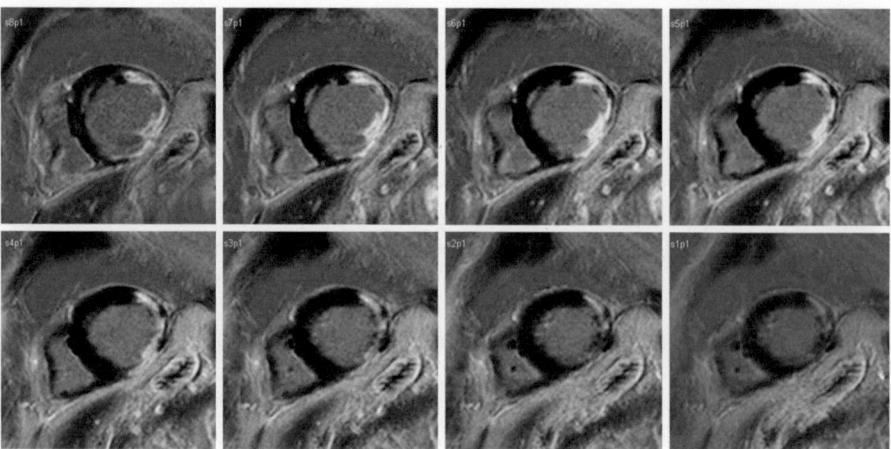

Fig. 1.17 Short-axis planes from an IR-TFE sequence obtained late after gadolinium administration showing delayed enhancement (*bright signal*) of the lateral left ventricular wall due to previous myocardial infarction

1.4.3.2 Practical Aspects of Obtaining Delayed Contrast Images

The waiting time of 10 min after administration of the contrast is necessary to allow it to wash out from the healthy ventricular myocardium. However, this interval is not necessarily wasted time, as it is possible to acquire the function study during this time, provided that the circulating contrast does not heavily affect the quality of the images from the *balanced TFE* sequences.

The number of slices in the *IR-TFE* sequence to acquire in each breath hold varies in relation to heart rate. It must be borne in mind that, if the apnoea is prolonged, the potential gain in speed will not compensate for the probable introduction of artefacts to the images if the patient does not maintain proper apnoea; it is preferable, for instance, to obtain two slices, each within an independent 10-s breath hold, than the same two slices in a 20-s apnoea, which the patient may be unable to maintain.

The optimal TI obtained from the *Look-Locker* sequence is not invariable; on the contrary, it tends to increase as time passes, which should be taken into account in cases of laborious acquisition of the delayed enhancement sequences.

1.4.3.3 Analysis of the Delayed Contrast Images

The areas of hyperintense myocardium (bright signal) which have retained gadolinium may be identified visually and correspond to scar tissue from either myocardial necrosis or fibrosis. On the other hand, segments of hypointense myocardium (dark signal), where contrast has been washed out, are considered healthy (non-scarred) heart muscle.

A semi-quantitative estimation can be performed of the delayed enhancement of ischemic origin (myocardial necrosis) by visual assessment of the level of transmurality of the scar tissue in a particular segment, which may be estimated as 0%

(absent), 1–25 % (strictly subendocardial), 26–50 %, 51–75 % and 76–100 % (practically transmural).

Similarly, it is also possible to make a quantitative evaluation of the extension of the delayed contrast by means of programmes that allow the analysis of the intensity of the myocardial signal and which identify myocardial necrosis (or fibrosis) in areas with an intensity of signal five times higher than the standard deviation from the mean obtained in an area of interest of the remote, healthy myocardium (see Fig. 1.18).

1.4.4 Study of Myocardial Perfusion

The study of myocardial perfusion consists of analysing the first pass of an intravenous injection of contrast (gadolinium) through the ventricular myocardium. For this, saturation recovery turbo field echo or echo-planar sequences are used for which several modification strategies exist, always aimed at obtaining T1 weighting of the signal and very short acquisition times that allow repeated acquisition of a series of slices within each cardiac cycle. The information sought with this type of study is the status of myocardial blood flow and, in particular, its possible changes after a pharmacological stress intervention.

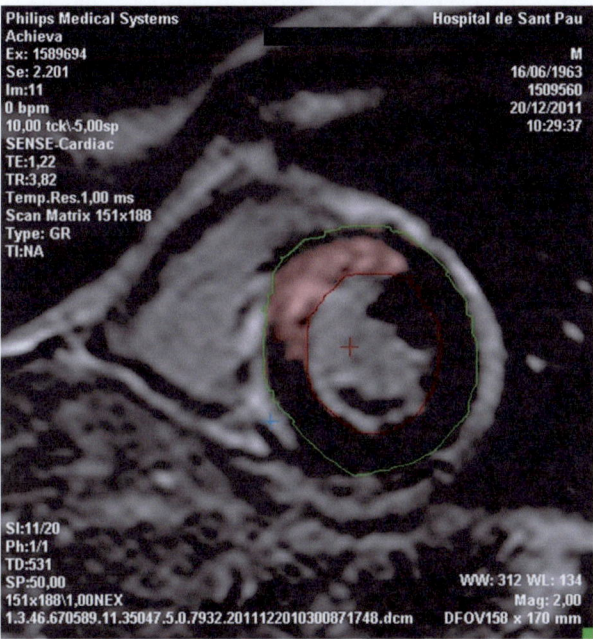

Fig. 1.18 Computer-aided detection of abnormal delayed contrast enhancement by deviation of signal intensity values with respect to those from remote healthy myocardium

1.4.4.1 Obtaining the Perfusion Images

The sequence is programmed with three parallel slices oriented on the ventricular short axis that are equidistant, with an interslice gap of 6–8 mm, centred approximately in the basal, medium and apical thirds of the left ventricle. The sequence is launched simultaneously with the quick injection of contrast (at 3–4 ml/s, ideally through an infusion bomb), in a dose of 0.075–0.1 mmol/kg, followed by 20–30 ml of saline solution at the same infusion speed.

The same process must be performed twice: at rest and 4 min after the administration of adenosine in continuous infusion at a dose of 140 µg/kg/min, as an agent of pharmacological stress. The effect of adenosine, as a potent vasodilator of the coronary arteries, is to increase blood flow in all myocardial areas dependent on non-obstructed vessels, while impaired perfusion is expected in those with significant coronary stenosis, in part as a result of steal phenomenon due to the increased blood flow in healthy regions. Between both acquisitions there must be a minimum interval of 10 min for the purposes of allowing some clearing of contrast from the circulation and the myocardium itself before the second acquisition.

1.4.4.2 Practical Aspects of Obtaining Perfusion Images

As the duration of the sequence is nearly 1 min, it is necessary to concentrate the patient's apnoea in the critical phase of the process, which is the arrival of contrast to the left ventricular myocardium (first pass). For this, we monitor, through a real-time display, the arrival of the contrast in the right cardiac chambers (see Fig. 1.19, upper row), a moment in which the patient is instructed to breathe in and then breathe out and hold his/her breath for as long as possible. This will probably allow for 15–20 s of apnoea which is enough for visualising the mentioned first pass of contrast through the left ventricular myocardium without respiratory interference (see Fig. 1.19, lower row).

The temporal resolution readout of each slice, of 100–125 ms, implies that, at high heart rates (>95–100 bpm), the three slices cannot be obtained within a single cardiac cycle. In these cases, the acquisition of the whole three slices is performed throughout two consecutive cardiac cycles. This represents a relative drawback, as is the slower sampling of the process of the first pass of contrast.

The norm is to carry out the adenosine perfusion sequence first, given that the images from a second acquisition may be somewhat less clear due to the residual circulating contrast from the first injection. Nevertheless, in patients with a prior myocardial infarction, we believe that it is recommendable to perform the basal study first with the aim of detecting the possible presence of fixed perfusion defects at rest.

1.4.4.3 Analysis of Perfusion Images

The study of myocardial perfusion is made qualitatively, by means of a comparative analysis of the sequences obtained at rest and during the administration of adenosine. The failure of any myocardial area to show increased signal relative to the rest of the myocardium during the first pass of the contrast is considered to be due a perfusion defect (see Fig. 1.1e). If this defect appears in the study with adenosine (arrows in the top row of images in Fig. 1.20), but not at rest (Fig. 1.20, lower row), it is considered to be an inducible perfusion defect.

1 Magnetic Resonance Sequences for Cardiovascular Applications and Study Planning 21

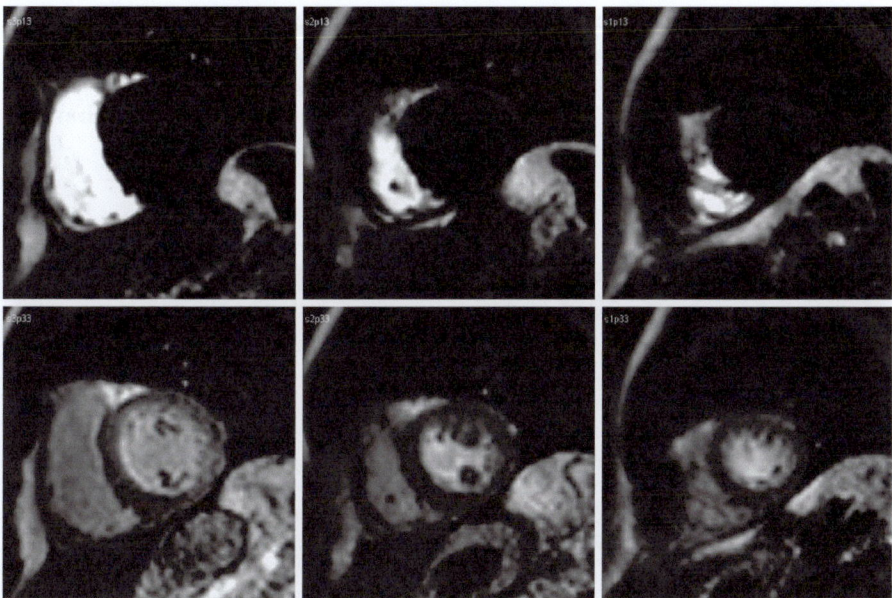

Fig. 1.19 Time course of the first pass of contrast through the cardiac chambers as visualised in the real-time viewer window. At the arrival of contrast to the right heart chambers (*upper panels*), the patient is asked to hold his/her breath in order to have a smooth set of images at the time of the first pass of contrast through the left ventricular myocardium (*lower panels*)

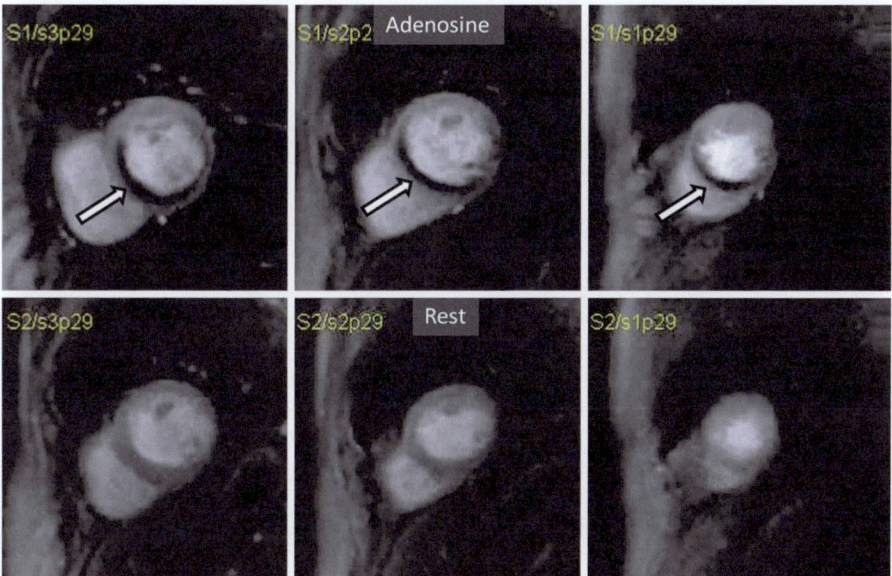

Fig. 1.20 Perfusion study showing an inducible defect (*arrows*) during adenosine infusion (*upper row*) which is not present in rest (*lower row*)

Software is available that analyses the intensity of the myocardial signal throughout the sequence, presenting curves of the ventricular segments in which it is possible to semi-quantify the state of perfusion by maximal amplitude or the slope of the curves (see Fig. 1.21). This is a cumbersome process, however, which means that it is not often used in practise.

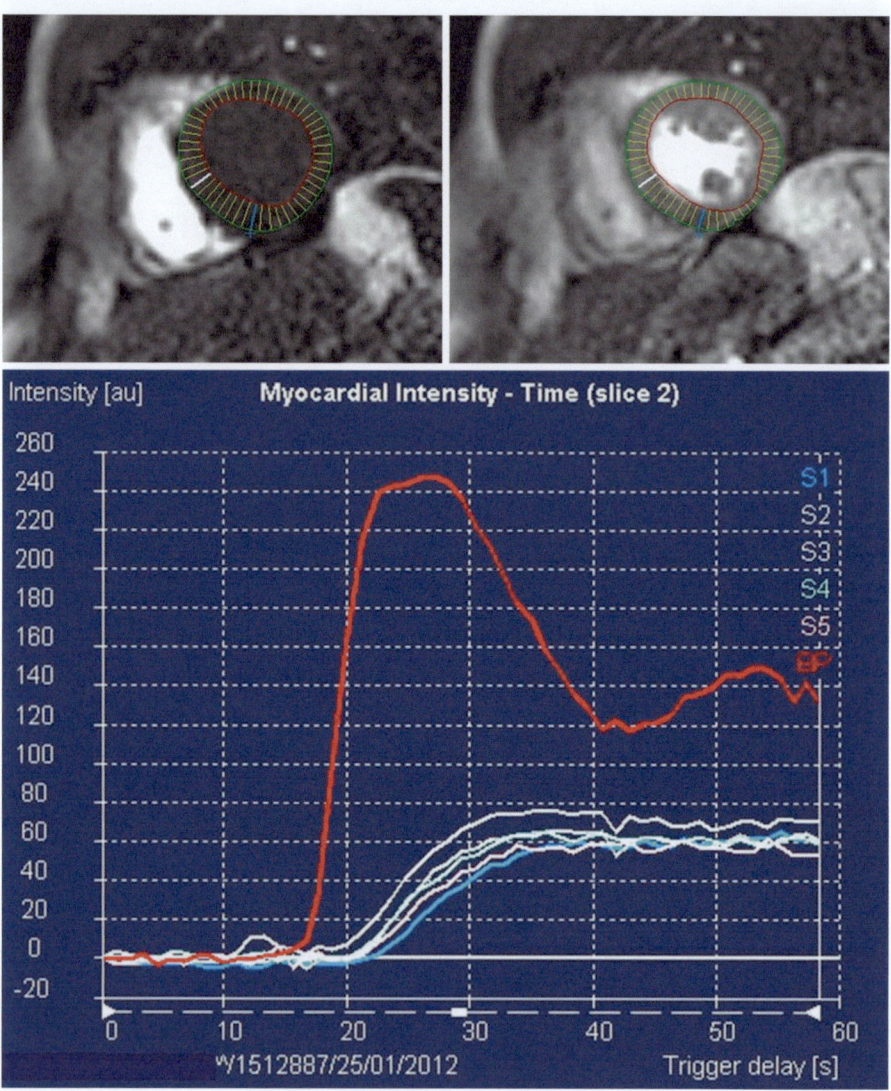

Fig. 1.21 Computer-aided analysis of myocardial first-pass perfusion by the time course of myocardial signal intensity at different segments from the study plane and, also, at the blood pool for reference (*lower panel*)

1.4.4.4 Practical Aspects of Perfusion Image Analysis

A relatively frequent problem is the presence of so-called "dark border" artefacts attributable to an effect of magnetic susceptibility in relation to the concentration of the contrast in the left ventricular cavity. This artefact is strictly limited to the subendocardial region, is almost completely linear and can simulate a genuine perfusion defect, although it is generally more transient. The visualisation of the same effect in the rest and stress studies favours its recognition as an artefact (arrows in Fig. 1.22) as long as there is no subendocardial necrosis, which must be checked, in turn, in the delayed contrast study.

1.4.5 Studies of Inducible Ischemia Based on Wall Motion Analysis

The strategy applied in this method is the acquiring of images of function (cine MR) by means of a *balanced TFE* sequence that is repeated through a series of steps of a protocol of increasing doses of dobutamine as a stress agent, in a similar way to stress echocardiography studies. The appearance of a segmental wall motion abnormality not present at rest is indicative of the induction of myocardial ischemia, the mechanism of which is an increase in oxygen demand caused by the dobutamine which cannot be met in this area due to the presence of a significant coronary artery stenosis.

1.4.5.1 Obtaining Ischemia Induction Studies by Wall Motion Analysis

Series of a *balanced TFE* sequence are programmed in three slices to be obtained in apnoea, oriented along the longitudinal axes of the two- and four-chamber views, as

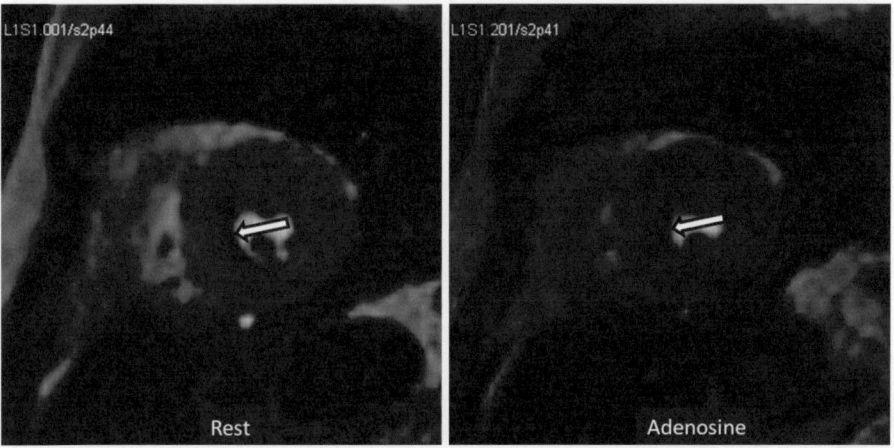

Fig. 1.22 First-pass perfusion study showing a "dark border" artefact not to be confused with an actual perfusion defect: being present at both rest (*left panel*) and stress (*right panel*) studies favours its artefactual nature

well as on a three-chamber plane, which includes the left ventricular outflow tract. As a complement to the latter, another acquisition to obtain three parallel slices in a second apnoea on the short ventricular axis at basal, mid- and apical levels is programmed. These six cine acquisitions are performed at rest and at the end of each step of the protocol with progressive doses of dobutamine: 5, 10, 20, 30 and 40 µg/kg/min. The duration of each step is 3 min.

1.4.5.2 Practical Aspects of Ischemia Induction Studies by Wall Motion Analysis

Precise control of the changes in heart rate and blood pressure at each step of the protocol is necessary. This requires monitoring equipment that is compatible with the magnetic field in the interior of the resonance room.

It is important to ensure that the heart rate has increased until at least 85 % of the theoretical maximum (220 minus age in years of the patient). If this value is not reached with 40 µg/kg/min of dobutamine, atropine may be administered in a dose of 0.5 mg by direct injection and may be repeated at intervals of 3 min up to a maximum dose of 1.5 mg.

Apart from reaching the maximal heart rate, the test may be prematurely concluded if the patient has presented with an induced segmental wall motion defect at an early stage, or if adverse effects from the dobutamine infusion are observed, such as repetitive ventricular arrhythmia or a significant hypertensive reaction.

1.4.5.3 Analysis of Wall Motion Studies of Ischemia Induction

The study of the images is carried out visually, by comparing slices at each stage side-by-side with the corresponding ones at rest. In order to detect a possible induction of segmental defects in stages prior to the maximum, a continuous analysis of the cine images after obtaining them at each level of stimulation is necessary. This requires a close inspection of end-systolic frames at each level of stimulation for the detection of induced regional hypokinesia (Fig. 1.23, arrows in the lower row).

1.4.6 Study of Blood Flow

The study of blood flow in large vessels is carried out with *phase contrast* sequences, which provide a map in which the direction of flow and velocity changes are encoded. This sequence can be oriented perpendicular to the vessel to be analysed, to obtain an instantaneous velocity profile (Fig. 1.24).

1.4.6.1 Obtaining Flow Images

In practice, we are mainly interested in the study of the flow of large vessels (aorta and pulmonary artery). The positioning of the slice is established, in the case of the aorta, on a coronal scout plane, with a strict axial orientation aligned with the level of the main pulmonary artery (see Fig. 1.25). The flow of the pulmonary artery requires an orientation with a double angulation: on one hand, on a sagittal plane at the level of the vessel (see Fig. 1.25, left) and also on an axial plane (see Fig 1.25,

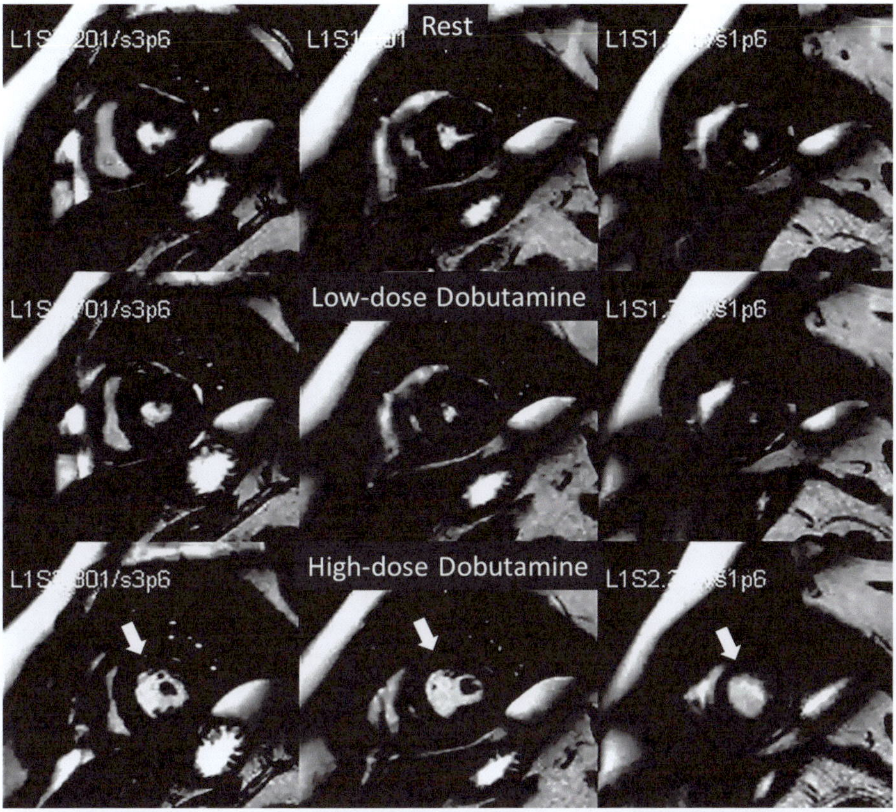

1 Magnetic Resonance Sequences for Cardiovascular Applications and Study Planning

Fig. 1.23 Series of end-systolic short-axis images from a stress dobutamine study showing marked dyskinesia of the anterior wall at the stage of maximal stimulation indicating inducible ischemia

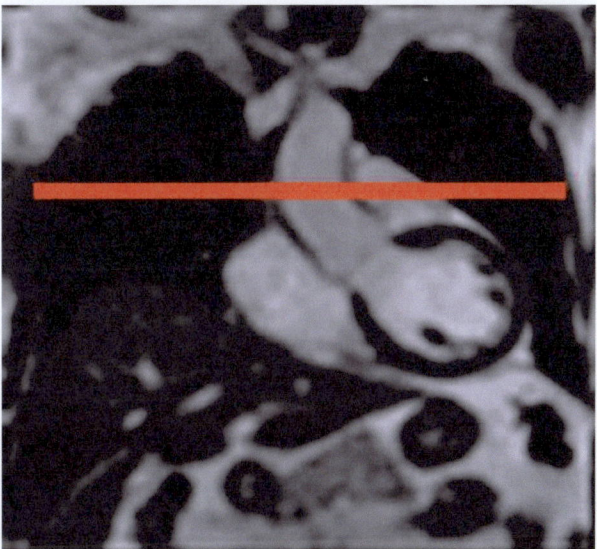

Fig. 1.24 Planning of a phase contrast study of the ascending aorta on a coronal scout plane

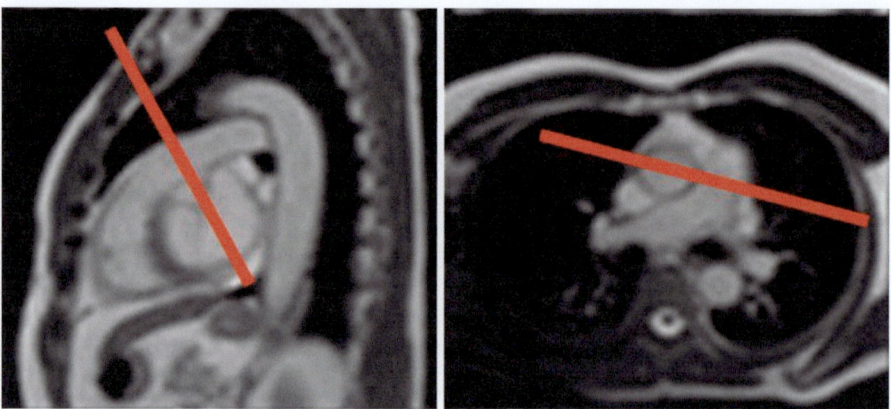

Fig. 1.25 Planning of a phase contrast study of the main pulmonary artery by double angulation on sagittal (*left panel*) and axial (*right panel*) planes where the vessel is visualised on longitudinal axis

right). The resulting images consist of two series of multiple phases from the cardiac cycle, one that is called the magnitude image, with the anatomical image as a reference, and one known as a phase image, with an encoding of the flow direction and velocities expressed as signal intensity changes within the vessel (see Fig. 1.1g).

1.4.6.2 Practical Aspects of Obtaining Flow Studies

Apart from a perfect transverse orientation of the vessel, a fundamental parameter in this kind of study is the velocity encoding (VENC), which determines the maximum velocity detectable for the codification and which must be adjusted to the real flow velocity; if the VENC is lower than the actual value, a fold-over of the information at the voxel level results, which gives rise to an artefact known as aliasing, which impedes the detection of the actual velocity and, therefore, the reconstruction of adequate flow curves. On the other hand, the higher the VENC is set, the more noise is introduced to the images, and the sensitivity to changes in velocity is reduced. The recommended VENC values of the pulmonary artery and aorta, in the absence of valvular stenosis, are around 150 and 200 cm/s, respectively. In the case of an aliasing phenomenon being identified in the velocity signal, the sequence must be repeated at a progressively higher VENC.

The velocity map sequences can be acquired in a period of apnoea or with a sequence of free respiration with respiratory synchronisation through a diaphragmatic navigator that monitors the movements of the diaphragm and limits the acquisition to a specific period of the respiratory cycle. In principle, this last modality allows a more accurate reading in the absence of arrhythmias.

1.4.6.3 Analysing Flow Images

Flow analyses are carried out at the workstation using the appropriate programme. It is necessary to trace or indicate the vessel in question to the equipment in the magnitude image, where its inner contours are automatically detected by the analysis programme, which extends them to all images in both the magnitude and phase acquisitions. With the information from the phase images, the equipment generates a curve of instantaneous blood flow throughout the cardiac cycle, in which it is possible to quantify the antegrade blood volume and, if present, a retrograde volume. The process can be performed on any vascular structure included in the plane as long as it is oriented orthogonally to the slice plane (see Fig. 1.26).

1.4.7 MR Contrast Angiography

This sequence (MR angiography) allows the acquirement of multiple parallel slices in a period of apnoea, during the passage of a contrast bolus through a segment of the large vessels, with which the stack of planes is oriented. Images can be reconstructed afterwards as a 3D volume with subtraction of the non-contrasted structures to highlight the signal from the vessel filled with contrast.

1.4.7.1 Obtaining the MR Angiogram Images

In the case, for example, of an angiogram of the thoracic aorta, the series of slices is oriented on an axial plane where the ascending and descending aorta is seen in an oblique sagittal angulation (see Fig. 1.27, left), taking particular care to include in the acquisition the whole extension of the thoracic aorta and of its upper abdominal segment through the adjustment of the slices along a localiser sagittal plane in which the vessel is visualised (see Fig. 1.27, right).

First, once the desired orientation is reached, a "mask" sequence is launched without injection of contrast, which will be subtracted from the sequence with contrast to suppress the non-contrasted structures and thus highlight the vessels. Next, a fast sequence is launched to follow the contrast injection, known as *2D bolus tracking*, in axial orientation, and a dose of 0.1 mmol/kg of a gadolinium compound

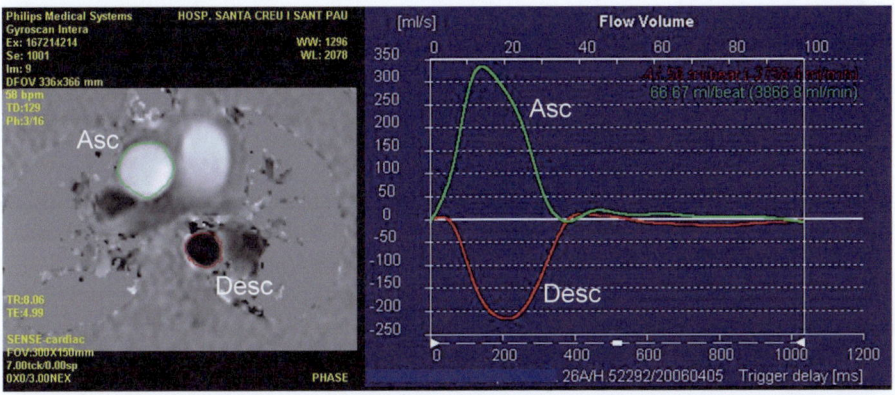

Fig. 1.26 Tracings of contours of the ascending and descending aorta on a phase contrast image (*left panel*) and the resultant flow curves (*right panel*)

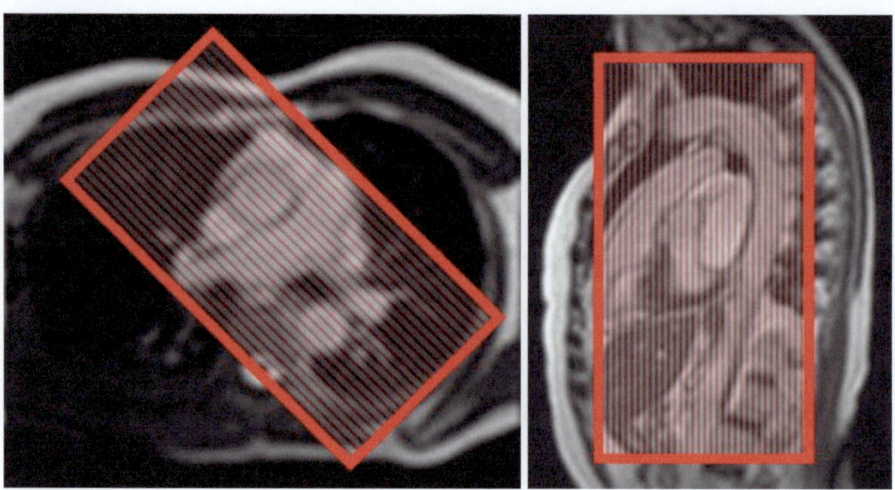

Fig. 1.27 Positioning of the stack of slices for an MR contrast angiography of the thoracic aorta on axial (*left panel*) and sagittal (*right panel*) scout images

is administered. At the moment when it is apparent in the *2D bolus tracking* sequence that the contrast completely fills the pulmonary artery tree (see boxed image in Fig. 1.28), the patient is instructed to start a breath hold, and the MR angiography sequence is launched.

1.4.7.2 Practical Aspects of Obtaining MR Angiogram Sequences
As a general rule, an MR angiography sequence requires a prolonged apnoea of 20–30 s. As interference from the respiratory movements notably degrades the images, it is important to instruct the patient to hold their breath for as long as possible and, also, to reduce the time of acquisition of the sequence to a minimum. This can be done by reducing the number of slices, which can be compensated by an increase of their width or, also, by reducing the acquisition matrix, although both interventions cause reduced spatial resolution. On the other hand, special techniques of k-space sampling (e.g. CENTRA) can be used, which make the sequences less sensitive to moving artefacts as the acquisition proceeds.

1.4.7.3 Analysing MR Angiogram Images
The MR angiogram may be analysed on slices reconstructed from the whole 3D data set with any orientation (see Fig. 1.1h) in the format of maximum intensity projection (MIP) (see Fig. 1.29, left) or a 3D rendering (see Fig. 1.29, right).

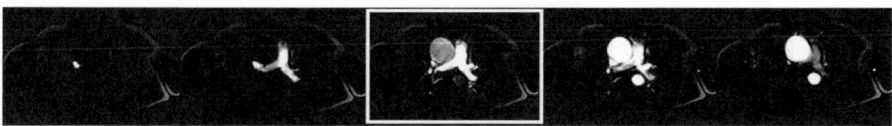

Fig 1.28 Time sequence of a bolus tracking technique during an MR contrast angiography as visualised on the real-time viewer window. The patient is instructed to hold his/her breath at the arrival of contrast to the pulmonary artery (*centre image*) to allow for a smooth set of images at the time of the filling of the aorta, when the sequence is launched

1.4.8 Study of Coronary MR Angiograms

The *whole-heart coronary MRA* sequence allows a series of multiple (100–120) parallel planes to be obtained, each of reduced thickness (1 mm), from which a 3D volume can be reconstructed with sufficient resolution to permit the analysis of the coronary arteries.

1.4.8.1 Obtaining the Coronary MR Angiogram Images

It is necessary to obtain a standard *balanced TFE* cine sequence in four-chamber orientation with high temporal resolution (up to 40 phases per cardiac cycle) to determine the longest interval when the position of the heart remains stable, which usually occurs during the diastolic phase and lasts for approximately 100 msec.

The *whole-heart* sequence is programmed in axial orientation beginning at the level of the main pulmonary artery, adjusting the delay at the start of the acquisition and its duration to the interval estimated in the previous cine sequence. The sequence is obtained without the administration of contrast, with free respiration, although with respiratory synchronisation through a diaphragmatic navigator (see Fig. 1.30) and often lasts between 5 and 10 min, depending on the efficiency of the navigator, which is why it is important to ensure that the patient maintains a regular pattern of respiratory movement.

1.4.8.2 Analysis of Coronary MR Angiogram Images

The volume obtained can be processed at a workstation, analysing the coronary vessel in the axial images themselves (see Fig. 1.31a), in a 3D reconstruction (see Fig. 1.31b) or from 2D multiplanar reconstructions (see Fig. 1.31c).

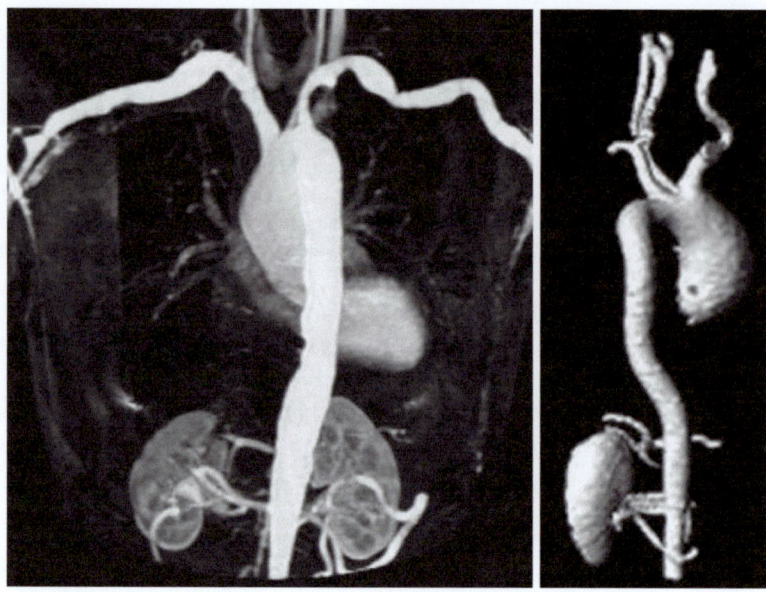

Fig. 1.29 MIP (*left panel*) and 3D rendering (*right panel*) of MR contrast angiography studies of the aorta

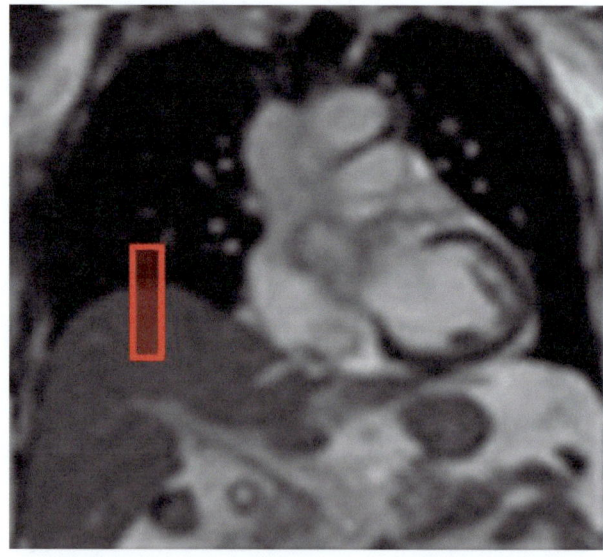

Fig. 1.30 Positioning of the diaphragmatic navigator on a coronal plane for obtaining a whole-heart study of the coronary arteries

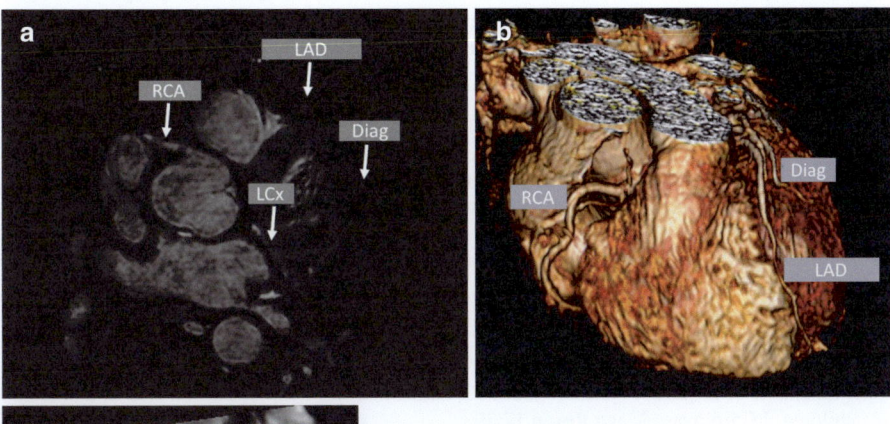
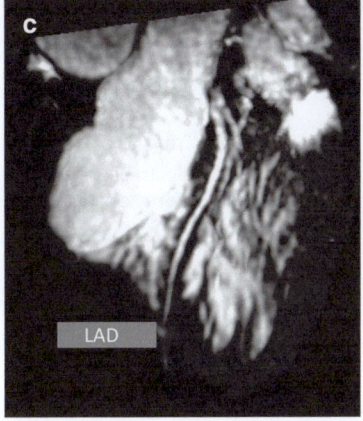

Fig. 1.31 Whole-heart sequence for the study of the coronary arteries. (**a**) Axial native plane; (**b**) 3D reconstruction; (**c**) multiplanar reconstruction. *Diag* diagonal artery, *LAD* left anterior descending, *LCx* left circumflex, *RCA* right coronary artery

Recommended Bibliography

1. Bitar R, Leung G, Perng R, Tadros S, Moody AR, Sarrazin J et al (2006) MR pulse sequences: what every radiologist wants to know but is afraid to ask. Radiographics 26:513–537
2. Cerqueira MD, Weissman NJ, Dilsizian V, Jacobs AK, Kaul S, Laskey WK et al (2002) Standardized myocardial segmentation and nomenclature for tomographic imaging of the heart: a statement for healthcare professionals from the Cardiac Imaging Committee of the Council on Clinical Cardiology of the American Heart Association. Circulation 105:539–542
3. Chiribiri A, Ishida M, Nagel E, Botnar RM (2011) Coronary imaging with cardiovascular magnetic resonance: current state of the art. Prog Cardiovasc Dis 54:240–252
4. Eitel I, Friedrich MG (2011) T2-weighted cardiovascular magnetic resonance in acute cardiac disease. J Cardiovasc Magn Reson 13:13
5. Friedrich MG, Bucciarelli-Ducci C, White JA, Plein S, Moon JC, Almeida AG et al (2014) Simplifying cardiovascular magnetic resonance pulse sequence terminology. J Cardiovasc Magn Reson 16:3960

6. Gerber B, Raman S, Nayak K, Epstein FH, Ferreira P, Axel L et al (2008) Myocardial first-pass perfusion cardiovascular magnetic resonance: history, theory, and current state of the art. J Cardiovasc Magn Reson 10:32
7. Hartung MP, Grist TM, François CJ (2011) Magnetic resonance angiography: current status and future directions. J Cardiovasc Magn Reson 13:19
8. Hundley WG, Bluemke D, Bogaert JG, Friedrich MG, Higgins CB, Lawson MA et al (2009) Society for Cardiovascular Magnetic Resonance guidelines for reporting cardiovascular magnetic resonance examinations. J Cardiovasc Magn Reson 11:5
9. Ibrahim EH (2011) Myocardial tagging by cardiovascular magnetic resonance: evolution of techniques-pulse sequences, analysis algorithms, and applications. J Cardiovasc Magn Reson 13:36
10. Kramer CM, Barkhausen J, Flamm SD, Kim RJ, Nagel E (2013) Standardized cardiovascular magnetic resonance (CMR) protocols 2013 update. J Cardiovasc Magn Reson 15:91
11. Kawel-Boehm N, Maceira A, Valsangiacomo-Buechel ER, Vogel-Claussen J, Turkbey EB, Williams R et al (2015) Normal values for cardiovascular magnetic resonance in adults and children. J Cardiovasc Magn Reson 17:29
12. Oshinski JN, Delfino JG, Sharma P, Gharib AM, Pettigrew RI (2010) Cardiovascular magnetic resonance at 3.0T: current state of the art. J Cardiovasc Magn Reson 120:55
13. Rodgers CT, Robson MD (2011) Cardiovascular magnetic resonance: physics and terminology. Prog Cardiovasc Dis 54:181–190
14. Schulz-Menger J, Bluemke DA, Bremerich J, Flamm SD, Fogel MA, Friedrich MG et al (2013) Standardized image interpretation and post processing in cardiovascular magnetic resonance: Society for Cardiovascular Magnetic Resonance (SCMR) board of trustees task force on standardized post processing. J Cardiovasc Magn Reson 15:35

CMR Study Protocol of Ischemic Heart Disease

2

Sandra Pujadas and Guillem Pons-Lladó

2.1 Introduction

Because of its numerous resources, Cardiovascular Magnetic Resonance (CMR) is the technique that offers greatest potential information on patients with ischemic heart disease. Its use is, therefore, a standard of reference in the study of ventricular volumes and function (global and segmental), and in the detection of myocardial necrosis; additionally, it has the capacity to characterise infarcted myocardial tissue and is also highly competitive among the different techniques of stress-induced ischemia. Nevertheless, it is not competitive nowadays for obtaining a non-invasive coronary angiogram, for which computed tomography is the technique of choice. But, overall, and leaving aside the study of the anatomy of the coronary arteries, CMR is the diagnostic modality that provides the most comprehensive information for the study of ischemic heart disease. Various strategies for its application should be considered, depending on the clinical situation. With this in mind, below we discuss a series of different diagnostic protocols.

2.2 Acute Myocardial Infarction (AMI)

The study protocol for a patient with an AMI is summarised in the following framework:

Sequence	Balanced TFE	STIR	T2*	Perfusion	Early IR TFE	Delayed IR TFE
Information	Ventricular function	Myocardial edema	Myocardial haemorrhage	Microvascular obstruction	Microvascular obstruction	Necrosis and viability

---

S. Pujadas, MD • G. Pons-Lladó, MD, PhD (✉)
Cardiac Imaging Unit, Cardiology Department, Hospital de la Santa Creu i Sant Pau,
Universitat Autònoma de Barcelona, Barcelona, Spain
e-mail: gpons@santpau.cat

2.2.1 Balanced FFE Cine: Ventricular Function Study

Following the protocol described in the previous chapter (see Chap. 1, Figs. 1.3, 1.4, 1.5, 1.6, and 1.7), cine sequences are performed on the vertical and horizontal planes, along with multiple short-axis cine series covering the whole extension of the heart. From these, calculations are made of the ventricular volumes and ejection fraction, as well as a careful analysis of the segmental wall motion (see Chap. 1, Figs. 1.8, 1.9, 1.10, and 1.11).

2.2.2 STIR Sequences: Myocardial Edema Detection

The presence of myocardial edema is an early and very sensitive sign of myocardial ischemia, whether or not the process has led to a myocardial necrosis. Given its transient nature, detecting or ruling out its presence is useful for establishing the chronology of a myocardial ischemic event. For this, T2-weighted TSE or STIR sequences along longitudinal and transversal planes of the heart (see Chap. 1, Fig. 1.14) are used, with the presence of myocardial edema being detected by increased signal intensity in the involved region. Based on the short-axis images, the area of myocardial edema can be traced (see Fig. 2.1., left panel). In the case of an AMI treated by primary angioplasty there is usually a difference between the extension of the myocardial edema, which indicates the area initially at risk, and that of the final necrosis. This difference, which it is possible to determine with CMR by comparing the STIR sequences with the delayed enhancement IR TFE ones (see Fig. 2.1, right panel), constitutes the so-called "salvaged myocardium". It is

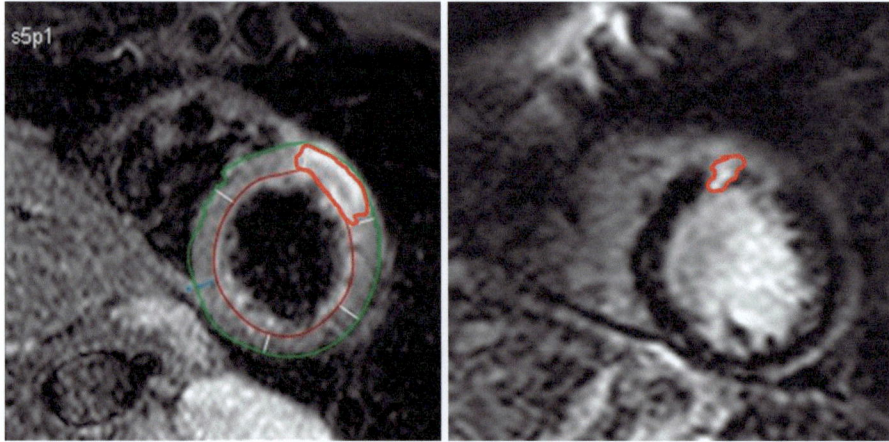

Fig. 2.1 Images from a STIR sequence (*left*) showing an area of increased signal intensity due to myocardial edema in a case of acute myocardial infarction treated by primary angioplasty, and the correspondent image from an Inversion Recovery sequence (*right*) with a much smaller area of delayed enhancement. The difference among them corresponds to myocardial tissue initially at risk but not actually infarcted (salvaged)

important to note that the study should be performed in the first week, as the myocardial edema is progressively reabsorbed afterwards.

2.2.3 T2* Sequences: Myocardial Haemorrhage

Extravasation of red blood cells may occur when reperfusion of an acute infarct is followed by a "no-reflow" phenomenon causing microvascular obstruction (MVO) and profound endothelial damage. The paramagnetic effects of haemoglobin degradation products are particularly strong when studied by T2*-weighted "Black-Blood" sequences, which are particularly sensitive to field inhomogeneities such as those caused by myocardial iron deposition or recent haemorrhage. Sequences are planned as a series of contiguous short-axis slices on which the presence of haemorrhage is detected by a signal void within the left ventricular myocardium (arrows, in Fig. 2.2).

2.2.4 Study of Rest Myocardial Perfusion: Detection of MVO

The study of the myocardial first pass of contrast in the case of an AMI allows the detection of perfusion defects due to MVO within the area of necrosis (see Fig. 2.3, arrow). The contrast dose (0.075–0.1 mmol/kg) and the planning of the slices are the usual for a perfusion study, as described in the previous chapter (see Chap. 1, Fig. 1.19). After the perfusion study, we proceed to inject the rest of the contrast (0.075–0.1 mmol/kg) in order that the subsequent sequences benefit from the full dose of contrast.

2.2.5 Early IR TFE Sequence: Detection of Microvascular Obstruction

Although the first-pass defect described is a sensitive sign of MVO, a more specific one is the persistence of a defective arrival of contrast. For this, 2 min after the contrast infusion, we acquire IR TFE sequences with the distinctive feature that, in this

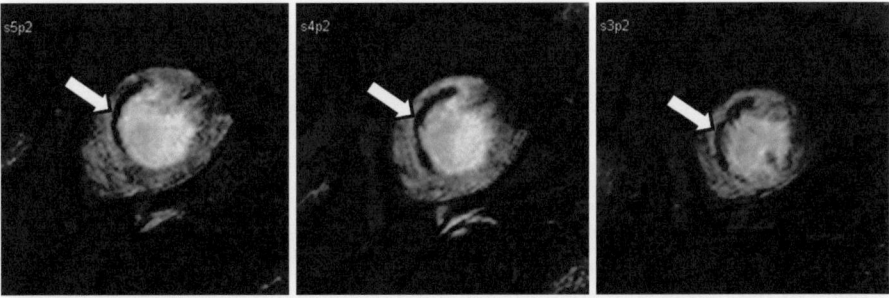

Fig. 2.2 Short axis slices from a Black-Blood T2* sequence in a patient with revascularized acute infarction showing an area of low signal intensity (*arrows*) due to intramyocardial hemorrhage

Fig. 2.3 First pass perfusion sequence in a patient with acute infarction showing a defect (*arrow*) suggestive of microvascular obstruction in the necrotic area

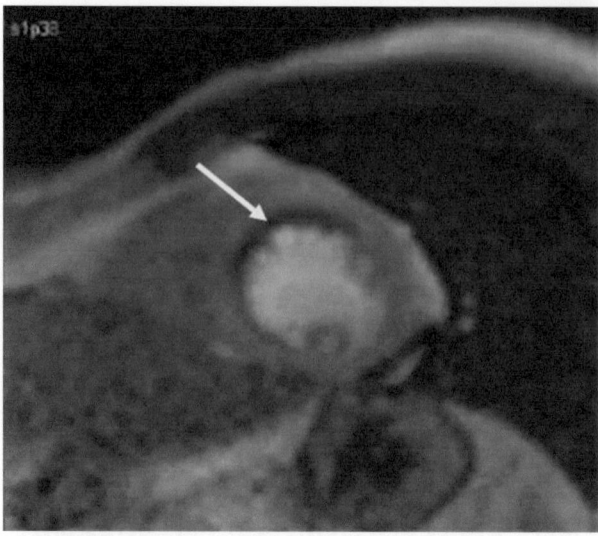

Fig. 2.4 IR TFE sequence acquired early (1–2 min) after the administration of contrast in a patient with acute infarction showing a region of low signal intensity indicating microvascular obstruction

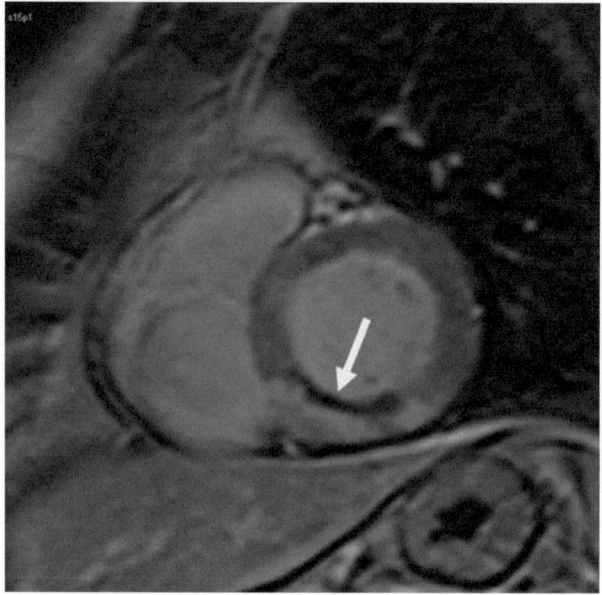

case, a long inversion time (400–600 ms) is applied, so that the signal from the healthy myocardium is not supressed but will, rather, show high signal intensity as a result of the presence of contrast, while the regions with microvascular obstruction – which the contrast cannot reach – will be shown with low signal intensity (see Fig. 2.4, arrow).

2.2.6 Delayed IR TFE Sequence: Study of Necrosis and Myocardial Viability

The delayed contrast enhancement sequence, applied by following the steps described in the previous chapter, with the corresponding adjustment of the inversion time in accordance with the *Look-Locker* sequence (see Chap. 1, Fig. 1.16), allows the area of myocardial necrosis to be visualised (see Chap. 1, Fig. 1.17) and its transmural extension to be determined. In practice, it is reported as <25 % (see Fig. 2.5, upper left panel), 25–50 % (see Fig. 2.5, upper right panel), 50–75 % (see Fig. 2.5, lower left panel) or 75–100 % or practically transmural (see Fig. 2.5, lower right panel). The significance of the residual viable myocardium is greater the lower the level of transmurality of the necrosis. An extension of scar tissue <50 % of wall

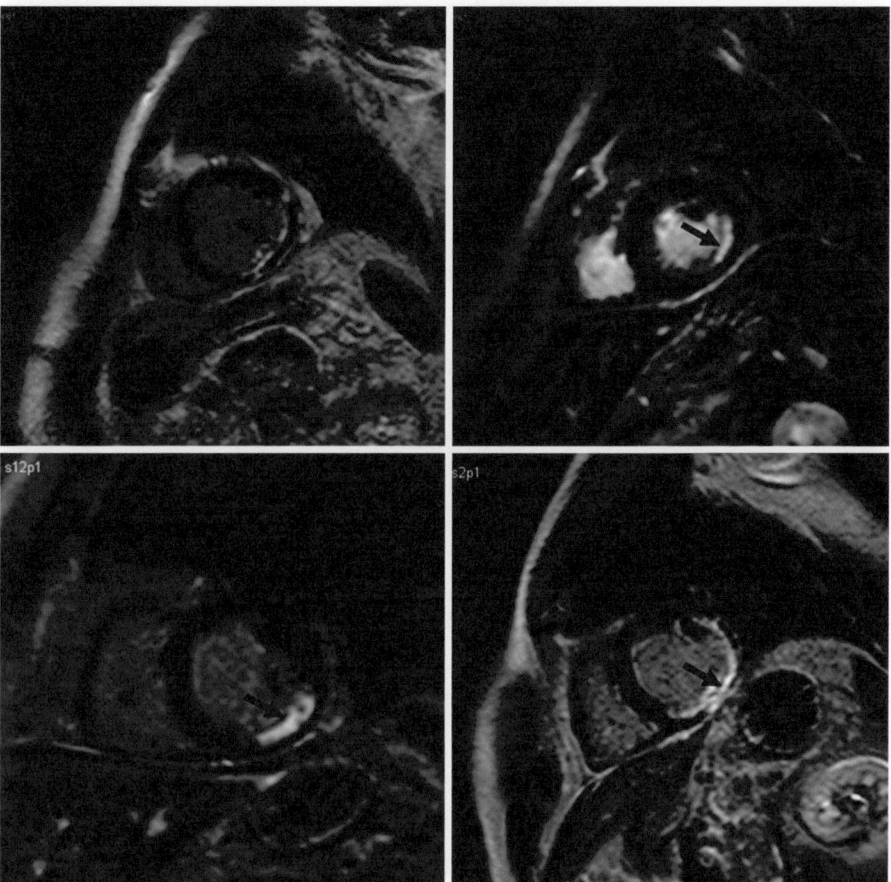

Fig. 2.5 Images from an IR TFE sequence acquired late (10 min) after contrast administration in four patients with lateral myocardial infarction showing different degrees of transmural involvement, from strictly subendocardial (*top left* image) to completely transmural (*bottom right* image)

Fig. 2.6 IR TFE sequence in a patient with recent infarction showing delayed contrast enhancement at the inferior wall with an area of low signal intensity within the infarcted region due to microvascular obstruction

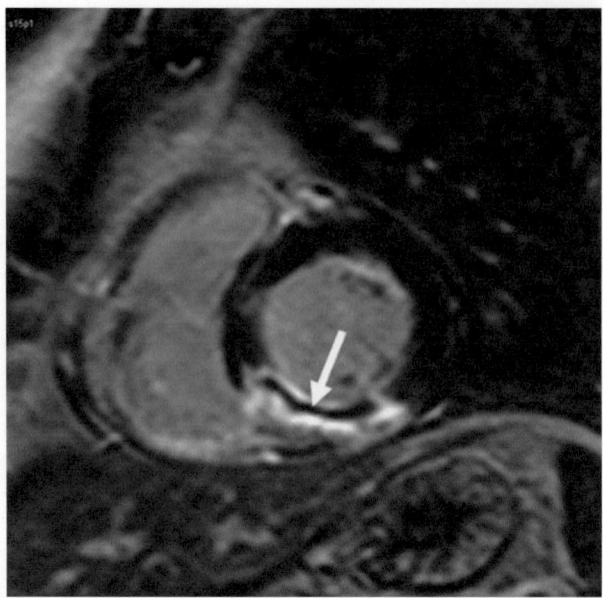

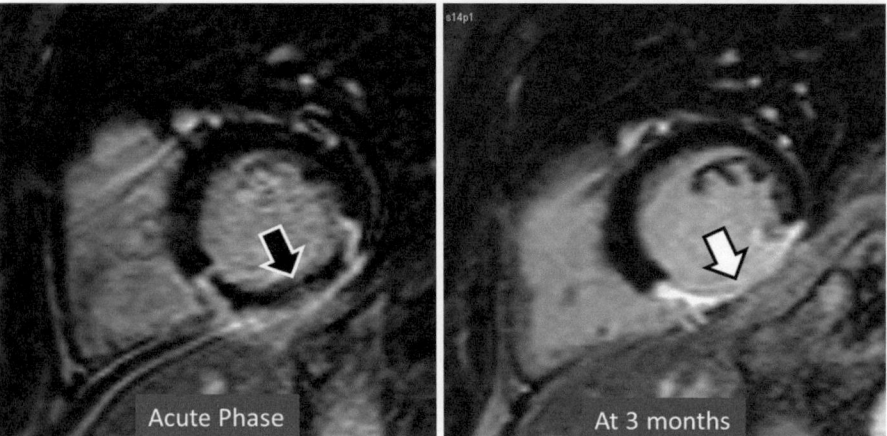

Fig. 2.7 Images from delayed enhancement studies on the same patient obtained early (*left panel*) and late (*right panel*) after infarction showing the evolution pattern from a necrosis with microvascular obstruction into an area of transmural compact scar with wall thinning

thickness is considered to be the cut-off point for the presence of potential myocardial viability and recovery of function after a successful revascularisation.

Again, in the case of AMI, the presence of MVO is also shown in this sequence by a region of low signal intensity within an area of myocardial necrosis (see Fig. 2.6, arrow).

It is worth noting that, once a case of AMI evolves into a subacute and, then, chronic state, CMR signs of edema and MVO (see Fig. 2.7, black arrow in left panel) disappear, the area of scar tissue is reduced and, in the case of transmural necrosis, the myocardial segment involved becomes thinner (see Fig. 2.7, white arrow in right panel).

2.3 CMR Studies with Pharmacological Stress

The detection of myocardial perfusion defects due to inducible ischemia by means of pharmacological stress is a CMR modality used to investigate suspected coronary artery disease, or, for patients in whom the condition has already been diagnosed, in order to assess its functional significance.

2.3.1 Stress CMR: Overview

The aim of the pharmacological stress study by CMR is to reveal the presence of functionally significant coronary stenosis and may be performed using a vasodilator agent causing hyperaemia (such as adenosine or dipyridamole) and first-pass perfusion sequences, or, alternatively, via a positive inotropic agent (such as dobutamine), the effect of which is evaluated through cine sequences to analyse contractile function. In the first case, an attempt is made to reveal a perfusion defect in the impaired myocardial area relative to the healthy regions. In the second modality, the aim is to demonstrate the induction of regional hypokinesia due to myocardial ischemia caused by the failure to meet elevated energy requirements because of insufficient supply.

Both modalities have demonstrated their diagnostic value, although in our group we consider perfusion studies with adenosine to be the first choice because they are faster, easier, and safer than dobutamine studies. Nevertheless, studies of function with dobutamine are an option in the case of contraindication for adenosine, or even for conditions not due to coronary atherosclerosis such as anomalous origin of coronary arteries or intramyocardial bridges for which a powerful inotropic stimulus is preferable to vasodilation for revealing the functional significance of the anomaly.

2.3.1.1 Required Equipment
- Monitoring equipment (blood pressure, cardiac rhythm and frequency and, ideally, pulse oximetry) compatible with the room's magnetic field.
- Cardiac arrest trolley.

2.3.1.2 Pharmacological Agents
- Adenosine (140 µg/kg/min for 6 min).
- Dobutamine (increasing doses, from 5 up to a maximum of 40 µg/kg/min).

2.3.1.3 Contraindications
- Adenosine:
    Known or suspected bronchospastic pulmonary disease
    Second or third-degree atrioventricular block

Sinus bradycardia (<45 bpm).
Systemic hypotension (<90 mmHg).
- Dobutamine:
  Severe hypertension (≥220/120 mmHg).
  Unstable angina.
  Severe aortic stenosis (area <1 cm^2, mean gradient ≥50 mmHg).
  Complex cardiac arrhythmia.
  Obstructive hypertrophic cardiomyopathy.
  Active myocarditis, pericarditis, or endocarditis.

2.3.1.4 Preparation of the Patient: Suppression of Prior Medication
- Adenosine: caffeine, theophylline and derivatives (coffee, tea, medications with caffeine, etc.) must be avoided for 24 h prior to the test.
- Dobutamine: beta-blocker and nitrate agent should be withdrawn 48 and 24 h previous to the test, respectively.

2.3.1.5 Possible Adverse Effects
- Adenosine: can cause flushing, precordial pain and palpitations. The most serious adverse effects include transitory atrioventricular block, hypotension, sinus tachycardia and acute bronchospasm.
- Dobutamine: can cause precordial pain, palpitations and hypertensive reaction. Although exceptional, cases of acute myocardial infarction, ventricular fibrillation and persistent ventricular tachycardia have been described.

2.3.2 CMR Study Protocols for Perfusion with Adenosine

The potential for a comprehensive body of information on the study of ischemic heart disease by CMR is fully exploited when the assessment of inducible ischemia by means of adenosine perfusion is regularly included in a complete protocol, alongside studies of function and delayed enhancement. The reason for this is the demonstrated greater diagnostic yield of the technique when information is obtained from the complete protocol rather than any of its parts. In the following framework the components of the protocol are detailed.

Sequence	Balanced TFE	Balanced TFE	Perfusion	Balanced TFE
Information	Two- and four-chamber cine: function	Short-axis cine (3 slices): pre-adenosine function	First pass of contrast during adenosine infusion	Short-axis cine (3 slices): function study during adenosine infusion

→	Balanced TFE	Perfusion	Waiting time (5 min)	DelayedIR TFE
	Multiple short-axis cine: function	First pass of contrast at rest		Necrosis and viability

2.3.2.1 Longitudinal and Pre-adenosine Short-axis Cine Sequence

As mentioned in the previous chapter, every CMR study begins with the acquisition of longitudinal cine sequences (see Chap. 1, Figs. 1.3, 1.4, 1.5, and 1.6), which also serve as localisers for the correct orientation of the planes in the rest of the study (see Fig. 1.7 of Chap. 1). In the case of the perfusion studies with adenosine we will also acquire a series of three equidistant cine slices oriented on the short axis, at basal, mid- and apical levels, coinciding with the position that will afterwards be used for the perfusion sequence. These cine sequences constitute the baseline study of regional wall motion to be compared with the same dataset obtained at the end of the adenosine infusion.

2.3.2.2 Perfusion Study with Adenosine

A perfusion sequence is planned, as indicated in Chap. 1, with three slices oriented on the ventricular short axis (see Chap. 1, Fig. 1.19). It is advisable to perform a first acquisition sequence of around 10 s without contrast injection to identify possible artefacts that may subsequently interfere with the analysis of the images. Once the suitability of the sequence is confirmed, the infusion of adenosine at the indicated dose (140 μg/kg/min) begins, with the patient outside of the magnet, checking the heart rate and blood pressure before the administration of the agent and regularly during the infusion. The objective of checking the constants is not only to ensure that there are no unwanted effects of adenosine, but also to confirm that it has had a proper vasodilatory effect, which can be inferred if a reduction in systolic blood pressure >10 mmHg is observed, and/or an increase in heart rate >10 bpm. In addition to this, the patient may also show symptoms of peripheral vasodilatation such as shortness of breath, chest discomfort, flushing, or headache, which also indicate an appropriate effect of the drug. Some patients, particularly the oldest ones, may present with an apparently blunted vasodilatory responsiveness at this dose of adenosine. If these signs and symptoms do not appear after 3 min of infusion, then the dose of adenosine is increased to 170 μg/kg/min for 2 min. If there is still no evidence of vasodilation, a final increase to 210 μg/kg/min for 2 more minutes can be performed. Most of the patients will respond to this high-dose scheme. Once the desired effect is obtained, and while the infusion is continued, the patient is placed inside the magnet again and the perfusion study begins.

The perfusion sequence is launched simultaneously with the injection of 0.075–0.1 mmol/kg of a gadolinium compound using an infusion pump at a speed of 3 ml/s, followed by the corresponding dose of saline solution. When we observe in the real-time viewer that the contrast has entered the right cardiac chambers, we instruct the patient to breath in, breath out, and then hold their breath for as long as they can manage, breathing gently afterwards until the end of the sequence, which usually takes 1 min to be completed. This ensures that there will be no respiratory interference at least during the acquisition of the images of the arrival (first pass) of the contrast to the ventricular myocardium.

The following framework summarises this acquisition process.

```
Start: continuous acquisition of images

         Injection of    Contrast
         contrast        arrives in
                         right ventricle

                                          Breath hold    Superficial breathing
                                          instruction
Time
─────────────────────────────────────────────────────────────────────────►
```

2.3.2.3 Adenosine Short-axis Cine Sequence

The same sequence of three short-axis cine slices obtained prior to the infusion of adenosine is repeated just after the perfusion sequence is completed, without interrupting the administration of the agent. These cines will be compared with those acquired at baseline in order to detect the appearance of induced defects in regional wall motion. This information is additional to the study of perfusion and indicative, when present, of particularly severe myocardial ischemia in the affected area (see Fig. 2.8, arrow in the right panel).

2.3.2.4 Multiple Short-axis Cine Sequence

The complete study of ventricular volumes and function is performed as described in the previous chapter (see Chap. 1, Fig. 1.7). The sequence is acquired at this point of the protocol to take advantage of the mandatory waiting time after the first perfusion to allow for the removal of the circulating contrast before the second perfusion is started, provided that, on the other hand, the presence of this circulating contrast does not essentially affect the quality of the SSFP sequences. Using this short-axis cine series it is possible to perform calculations of volumes and right and left ventricular ejection fraction, as well as analysing regional motion, as discussed previously (see Chap. 1, Figs. 1.8, 1.9, and 1.10).

2.3.2.5 Rest Perfusion Study

The first pass perfusion study is repeated in the "rest" state, ideally 15 min after adenosine acquisition. The sequence is programmed by copying that of the stress perfusion study (keeping the parameters and slice positions of the sequence unchanged), so that they may be compared later. In the analysis of the images, perfusion defects that appear in the stress study and not in the rest one are considered to be induced by the action of the adenosine (see Fig. 2.9, arrows), while the apparently "fixed" defects, meaning those that appear in the basal situation and in stress, in the absence of necrosis in the mentioned areas,

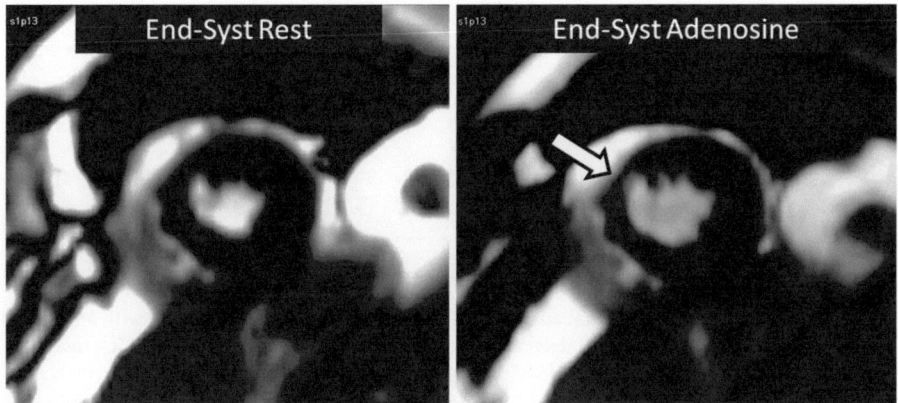

Fig. 2.8 End-systolic images from cine studies obtained at rest (*left*) and during adenosine (*right*) showing a stress-induced wall motion abnormality of the anterior wall (*arrow*)

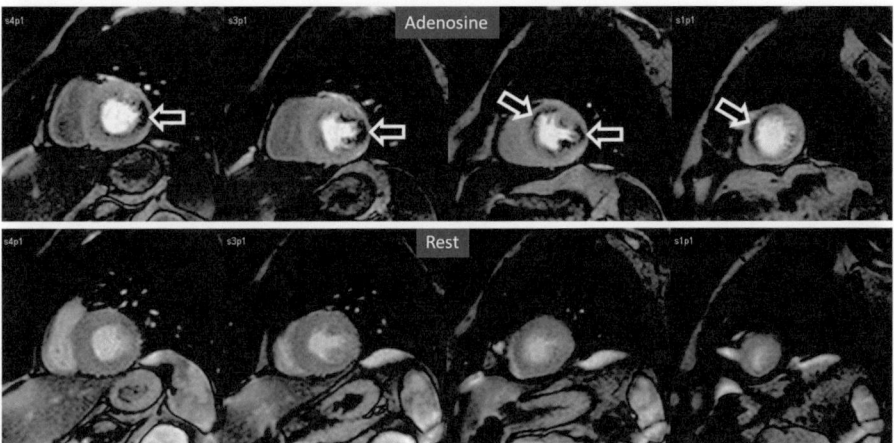

Fig. 2.9 Perfusion study showing extensive transmural defects induced by adenosine (*arrows*, in the *upper row* images) at the basal and middle lateral wall and at the mid-ventricular and apical antero-septal segments, none of them present at rest (*lower row*). The study indicates significant obstructive lesions of the left anterior descending and circumflex coronary arteries

are considered to be due to artefacts, as mentioned in the previous chapter (see Chap. 1, Fig. 1.22).

In the case of known prior myocardial infarction, in our group we prefer to invert the order of the perfusion studies and perform the rest study first. This is because, with a prior infarction, it is particularly important to identify possible increases in the area of the defect induced by adenosine. In the first-pass perfusion, this is unpredictable, particularly in the case of chronic infarcts. A baseline study to use as a reference is then useful. Performing the stress perfusion study second may cause it to suffer from the presence of contrast remaining from the rest study

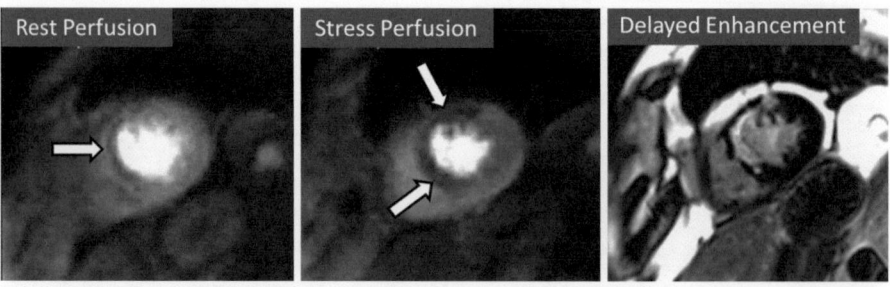

Fig. 2.10 Rest and stress perfusion and delayed enhancement studies in a patient with anteroseptal infarction. A fixed perfusion defect exists at rest (*arrow*, in the *left panel*), which increases in size at stress (*arrows*, in the *central panel*) corresponding to peri-infarction inducible ischemia, which is also supported by comparing the stress image with the delayed enhancement sequence (*right panel*), where the area of perfusion defect at stress is seen to exceed the one of the scarred tissue

in areas of necrosis, which may falsely normalise the perfusion in these otherwise infarcted regions, but the appearance of new areas of defective perfusion should be clearly distinguished by comparison of both studies (see Fig. 2.10, arrows in left and central panels). In any case, checking the delayed enhancement images for the actual extension of the area of necrosis would also be helpful (see Fig. 2.10, right panel).

2.3.2.6 Study of Delayed Contrast Enhancement

As the contrast used in the perfusion studies adds up to a total dose of 0.15–0.2 mmol/kg, we may now proceed to complete the protocol with a delayed contrast enhancement study, even if there is no clinical suspicion of prior infarction. For this, the *IR TFE* sequences set out in Chap. 1 apply, with a time gap of at least 5 min following the last administration of contrast.

2.3.3 CMR Study Protocol for Induction of Ischemia with Dobutamine

The studies using dobutamine as a stressor agent follow the protocol below:

Sequence	Balanced TFE	Balanced TFE	Perfusion	Balanced TFE
Information	2-and 4-chamber cine: function	Multiple short-axis cine: function	First pass at rest	Dobutamine at increasing doses

→	Perfusion	Waiting time (10 min)	Delayed IR TFE
	First pass under dobutamine		Necrosis and viability

2.3.3.1 Multiple Longitudinal and Short-axis Cines

In this case a full study of ventricular volumes and function is performed according to the protocol described in Chap. 1 before beginning with the pharmacological stimulation.

2.3.3.2 Perfusion Study at Rest

A study of myocardial perfusion at rest is obtained as usual (see Chap. 1, Fig. 1.19) with a dose of 0.75–0.1 mmol/kg of gadolinium.

2.3.3.3 Function Study with Dobutamine

Cine series of three slices are programmed oriented along the short and long axes (see Chap. 1, Fig. 1.23), which are acquired in two different breath holds (one for every series of three cines). These acquisitions will be repeated at the end of each stage of stimulation with dobutamine, which begins with a dose of 5 µg/kg/min and is increased every 3 min to 10, 20, 30 and finally 40 µg/kg/min. The infusion is performed with the patient inside the magnet and requires strict monitoring of the blood pressure and heart rate, as well as being attentive to the possible presentation of symptoms. In the case of not reaching 85 % of maximum theoretical heart rate (220 minus age of patient in years) with the dose of 40 µg/kg/min, 0.5 mg of direct atropine should be administered, repeated after 2 min if the desired frequency is not reached, up to a maximum dose of 1.5 mg.

The analysis of the function studies during stimulation aims to detect induced regional wall motion abnormalities with increasing doses of dobutamine. For this, it is particularly useful to examine the end-systolic phases of each stage, in which the hypokinesia induced may be assessed (see Fig. 2.11, arrow).

2.3.3.4 Perfusion Study with Dobutamine

Although not strictly necessary in a study of ischemia induction by dobutamine stimulation, if the patient has shown an adequate tolerance of the procedure, and given that the study must be completed with the delayed contrast enhancement sequences, it is reasonable to acquire a perfusion sequence during maximal dobutamine stimulation, again by giving a dose of 0.75–0.1 mmol/kg of gadolinium. The information

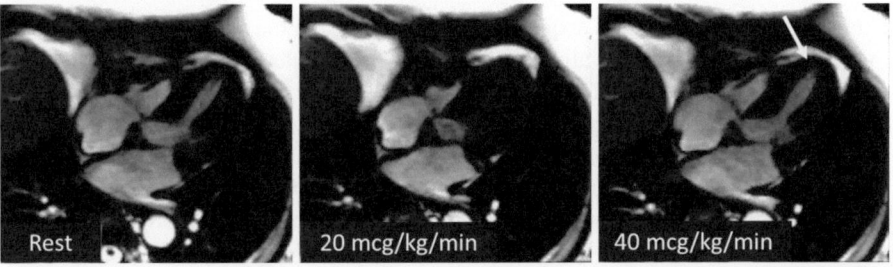

Fig. 2.11 Series of end-systolic four-chamber images from a stress dobutamine study showing dyskinesia of the septal and apical wall at the stage of maximal stimulation (*arrow*, in the *right panel*) indicating inducible ischemia

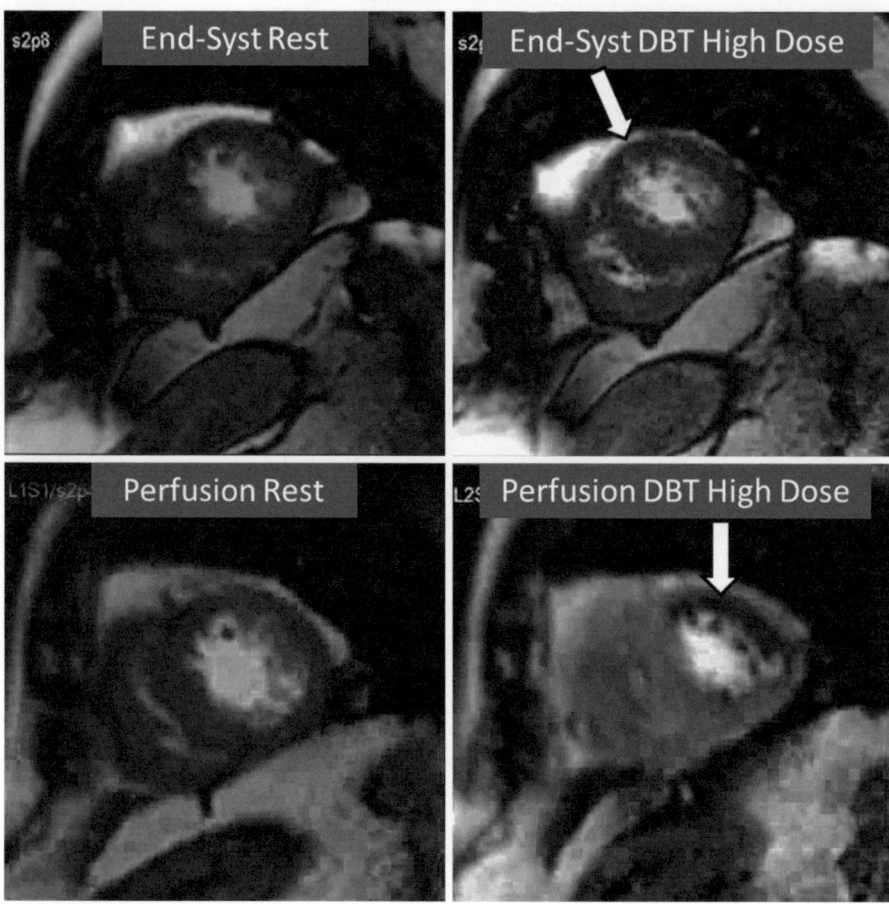

Fig. 2.12 End-systolic short axis frames (*upper row panels*) showing inducible wall motion abnormality at high dose dobutamine (*arrow*) which is corresponded by an stress induced defect of the same territory in the first pass perfusion sequence (*arrow, lower row*)

obtained from the perfusion sequences will complement the studies of function during dobutamine stimulation allowing the detection of a perfusion defect at maximal stimulation (see Fig. 2.12, arrow in bottom right panel) in addition to an induced wall motion abnormality (see Fig. 2.12, arrow in top right panel).

2.3.3.5 Study of Delayed Contrast Enhancement
This is performed as the last step, following the previously-described protocol.

2.4 Function and Viability Study

A number of patients with ischemic cardiomyopathy, especially those with multi-vascular disease, present with one or more previous episodes of necrosis and the subsequent left ventricular dysfunction involving more or less extensive myocardial

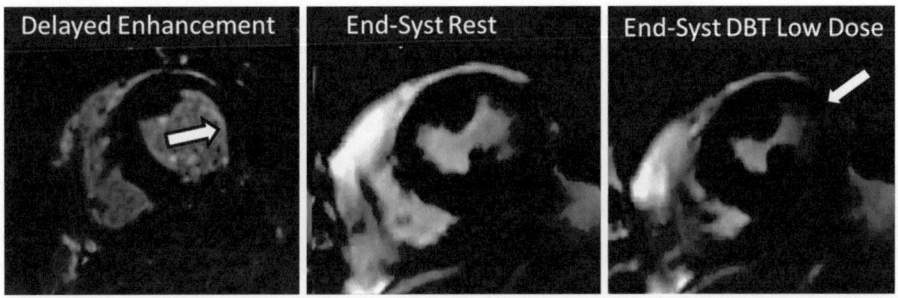

Fig. 2.13 Non-transmural (50%) myocardial infarction of the lateral wall in the delayed enhancement study (*arrow, left panel*), with end-systolic frames at the same level both at rest (*central panel*) and during dobutamine stimulation at low doses, showing increase in wall motion and thickening (*arrow, right panel*), this indicating the presence of contractile reserve in the involved segment

territories. The clinical question in these cases is the likelihood of potential recovery of function after revascularisation, which depends on the so-called "myocardial viability" of the impaired regions. Useful in this sense is the study of global and regional function, and the information from the delayed enhancement study, particularly on the degree of transmurality of necrosis. The study adjusts thus to the steps of the following framework.

Sequence	Balanced TFE	Balanced TFE	Delayed IR TFE	Balanced TFE
Information	Two- and four-chamber cine: function	Multiple short-axis cine: function	Necrosis and viability	Dobutamine at low dosage

The function and delayed contrast sequences are performed according to the protocols already mentioned. The addition of a function sequence under stimulation with dobutamine at low dosage (5, 10 and 20 µg/kg/min) may be considered where areas are shown of delayed contrast enhancement with transmural extension of around 50% (see Fig. 2.13, arrow in left panel). The demonstration of the presence of contractile reserve (i.e.: an increase in myocardial wall thickening with low-dose dobutamine) in a particular region (see Fig 2.13, arrow in right panel) is an additional argument in favour of myocardial viability in this area.

Recommended Bibliography

1. Gebker R, Jahnke C, Manka R, Hucko T, Schnackenburg B, Kelle S et al (2011) The role of dobutamine stress cardiovascular magnetic resonance in the clinical management of patients with suspected and known coronary artery disease. J Cardiovasc Magn Reson 13:46
2. Gerber B, Raman S, Nayak K, Epstein FH, Ferreira P, Axel L et al (2008) Myocardial first-pass perfusion cardiovascular magnetic resonance: history, theory, and current state of the art. J Cardiovasc Magn Reson 10:32
3. Kim HW, Farzaneh-Far A, Kim RJ (2010) Cardiovascular magnetic resonance in patients with myocardial infarction. Current and emerging applications. J Am Coll Cardiol 55:1–16

4. Mather AN, Lockie T, Nagel E, Marber M, Perera D, Redwood S et al (2009) Appearance of microvascular obstruction on high resolution first-pass perfusion, early and late gadolinium enhancement CMR in patients with acute myocardial infarction. J Cardiovasc Magn Reson 11:33
5. Perazzolo Marra M, Lima JA, Iliceto S (2011) MRI in acute myocardial infarction. Eur Heart J 32:284–293
6. Romero J, Xue X, Gonzalez W, Garcia MJ (2012) CMR imaging assessing viability in patients with chronic ventricular dysfunction due to coronary artery disease. J Am Coll Cardiol Img 5:494–508
7. Schwitter J, Arai A (2011) Assessment of cardiac ischaemia and viability: role of cardiovascular magnetic resonance. Eur Heart J 32:799–809
8. Ubachs JFA, Engblom H, Erlinge D, Jovinge S, Hedström E, Carlsson M et al (2010) Cardiovascular magnetic resonance of the myocardium at risk in acute reperfused myocardial infarction: comparison of T2-weighted imaging versus the circumferential endocardial extent of late gadolinium enhancement with transmural projection. J Cardiovasc Magn Reson 12:18
9. Wu KC (2012) CMR of microvascular obstruction and hemorrhage in myocardial infarction. J Cardiovasc Magn Reson 14:68

CMR Study Protocol of Cardiomyopathies

3

Sandra Pujadas and Guillem Pons-Lladó

3.1 Introduction

Cardiovascular magnetic resonance (CMR) is the leading technique for the study of ventricular volumes and function, which is fundamental information for the diagnosis and monitoring of patients with cardiomyopathy. Nevertheless, what has really made this technique unique in the study of heart muscle disease is its capacity to identify focal myocardial fibrosis. This information is helpful in determining the aetiology of the myocardial dysfunction and has implications for prognosis. The most common study protocol is quite simple and includes studies of function and delayed contrast enhancement as indicated in the following framework.

Sequence	*Balanced TFE*	*Balanced TFE*	*Delayed IR TFE*
Information	Two-, three- and four-chamber cine: function	Multiple short-axis cine: function	Necrosis and/or focal fibrosis

3.2 Dilated Cardiomyopathy

The clinical suspicion of dilated cardiomyopathy and the detection by echocardiography of left ventricular dysfunction of unclear origin are frequent causes for ordering a CMR study, for the reasons discussed above.

S. Pujadas, MD • G. Pons-Lladó, MD, PhD (✉)
Cardiac Imaging Unit, Cardiology Department, Hospital de la Santa Creu i Sant Pau,
Universitat Autònoma de Barcelona, Barcelona, Spain
e-mail: gpons@santpau.cat

3.2.1 Balanced FFE Cine: Ventricular Function Study

Following the protocol described in the first chapter (see Chap. 1, Figs. 1.3, 1.4, 1.5, 1.6 and 1.7), cine sequences on the vertical and horizontal planes are acquired, along with multiple cine series covering the whole extension of the heart. As explained, this constitutes the basis for calculating the ventricular volumes and the ejection fraction and assessing the regional wall motion patterns (see Chap. 1, Figs. 1.8, 1.9, 1.10 and 1.11).

3.2.2 Delayed IR TFE Sequence: Study of Necrosis and/or Focal Myocardial Fibrosis

The delayed enhancement sequence is performed following the steps described in Chap. 1, with the corresponding adjustment of the inversion time according to the *Look-Locker* sequence (see Chap. 1, Fig. 1.16). This sequence provides important information for the differential diagnosis of cardiomyopathies. Cardiomyopathies of ischaemic origin show delayed enhancement of variable extension, including either the whole wall thickness of a segment (transmural) or its subendocardial region (non-transmural). This finding indicates the presence of a myocardial scar of ischaemic origin (see Fig. 3.1, arrows in the left-hand panel), whether or not the patient has a clinical history of myocardial infarction. On the other hand, a proportion of patients with non-ischaemic cardiomyopathy do not show delayed enhancement, and when it occurs, which happens in approximately two thirds of cases, it shows a linear or focal intramyocardial pattern that spares the subendocardial region, which in this case is attributed to myocardial non-ischaemic fibrosis (see Fig. 3.1, arrow on right-hand panel). The finding of delayed enhancement of non-ischaemic origin, particularly when distributed as midwall striae, is a predictor of serious ventricular arrhythmias and sudden death in these patients.

3.3 Hypertrophic Cardiomyopathy

CMR has become a widely used technique for the diagnosis and prognostic stratification of hypertrophic cardiomyopathy. On the one hand, through the MR cine sequences, we can precisely define the anatomical distribution of the process and its phenotype and perform a precise measurement of the wall thickness in all ventricular segments. This is very useful in cases with atypical distribution of hypertrophy (arrows in Fig. 3.2), which may go unnoticed with echocardiography. On the other hand, the possibility of identifying the presence of focal intramyocardial fibrosis and its extension is an aspect of the technique of great interest, as it allows the anatomical diagnosis to be complemented by tissue information, which has been shown to have prognostic stratification value.

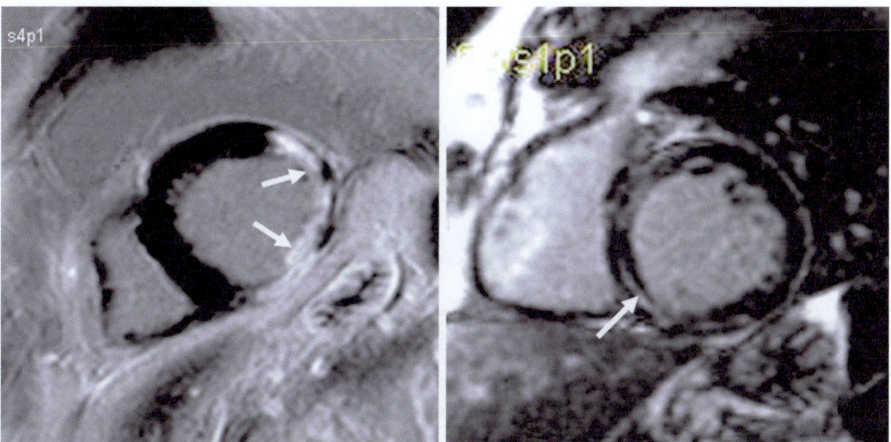

Fig. 3.1 IR TFE sequences showing delayed contrast enhancement (*arrows*) in a case of myocardial scarring of ischaemic origin (*left panel*) and in a patient with non-ischaemic cardiomyopathy (*right panel*)

Fig. 3.2 SSFP image in four-chamber view showing asymmetrical hypertrophy involving the midventricular region (*arrows*)

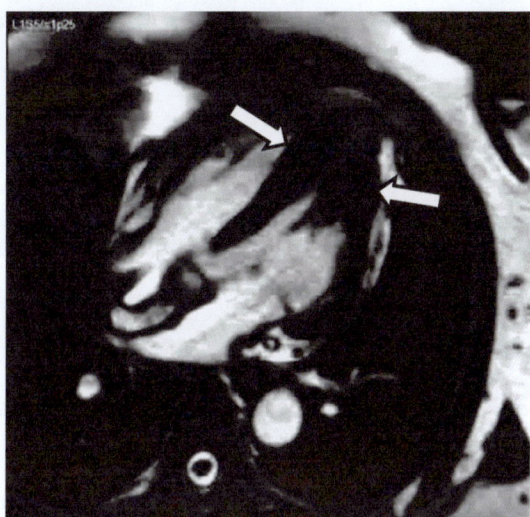

3.3.1 Balanced FFE Cine: Ventricular Function Study

The protocol is the same as that described for dilated cardiomyopathy, but with the addition of a longitudinal three-chamber plane that allows us to detect whether there is turbulent flow in the left ventricular outflow tract, which suggests a dynamic obstruction at this level (see Fig. 3.3, white arrow), and to assess the presence of systolic anterior motion of the mitral valve (see Fig. 3.3, black arrow).

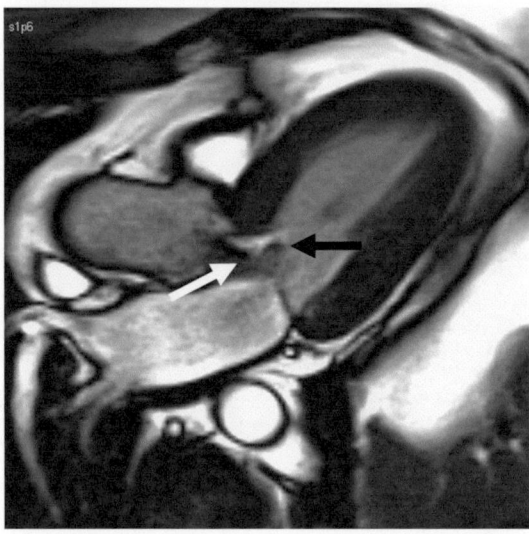

Fig. 3.3 Systolic frame from an SSFP cine sequence in a case of hypertrophic cardiomyopathy showing systolic anterior movement of the mitral valve (*black arrow*). There is also evidence of turbulent flow (*white arrow*) indicating obstruction at the left ventricular outflow tract

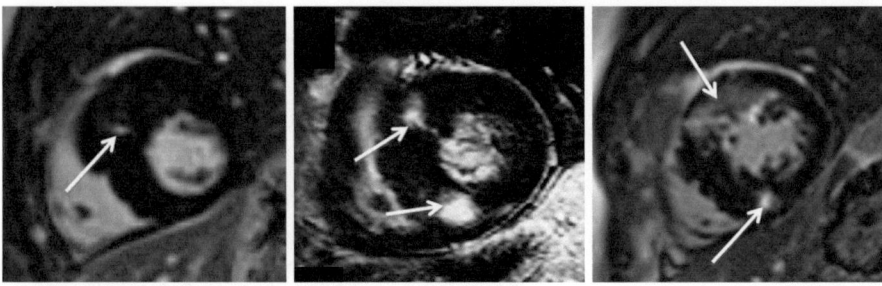

Fig. 3.4 IR TFE sequences showing delayed contrast enhancement (*arrows*) of different degree in three patients with hypertrophic cardiomyopathy

3.3.2 Delayed IR TFE Sequence: Study of Necrosis and/or Focal Myocardial Fibrosis

The delayed enhancement sequence is obtained according to the protocol described (see Chap. 1) and allows the identification, in up to two thirds of patients with hypertrophic cardiomyopathy, of regions of intramyocardial fibrosis. This presents in the form of midwall focal or patchy distribution. It may vary in extension and frequently involves the intraventricular septum in the regions of insertion of the right ventricular wall (see Fig. 3.4, arrows). This generally occurs in hypertrophied segments, but in advanced cases, it may also extend to areas with normal wall thickness as well (Fig. 3.5, left panel). There is evidence that the presence and extension of the intramyocardial fibrosis in hypertrophic cardiomyopathy are markers of poor prognosis, both in terms of evolution of the process towards a remodelled left ventricle, with progressive systolic dysfunction, and the presentation of potentially serious

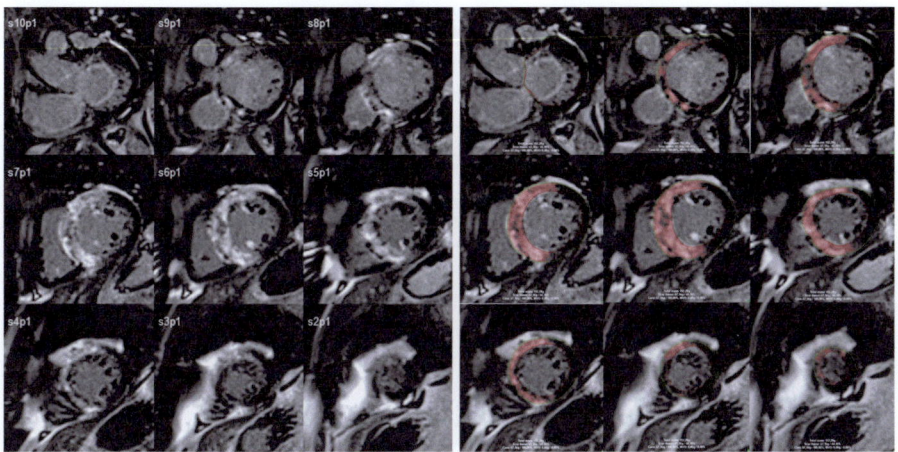

Fig. 3.5 IR TFE sequence showing extensive delayed contrast enhancement in a patient with hypertrophic cardiomyopathy (*left panel*) and its quantitative assessment by computer detection of the enhanced myocardium (*right panel*)

arrhythmias. The measurement of the fibrotic area may be performed similarly to the calculation of the mass of scar tissue in myocardial infarction (Fig. 3.5, right panel). It has been reported that a value >15 % of the total left ventricular mass may constitute a primary risk marker for sudden death in this disease. Although still under study, the presence and extent of intramyocardial fibrosis in hypertrophic cardiomyopathy may provide useful additional information for decisions on preventive measures in patients with ambiguous risk status based on conventional risk factors.

3.4 Left Ventricular Noncompaction

The phenotype of this genetic cardiomyopathy exhibits an extensive network of myocardial trabeculation and is interpreted as a defect in the normal development of the process of foetal myocardial compaction. Frequently it is associated with systolic dysfunction and ventricular dilation, which are determinant prognostic factors. The fact that it may appear in the absence of ventricular dysfunction, as well as the relative prominence of intraventricular trabeculae in otherwise normal hearts, means that its diagnosis is frequently uncertain. The echocardiographic suspicion of a compaction defect is a common cause of request for a CMR study.

The basic CMR protocol (function and delayed enhancement) is applied, and the required diagnostic criteria are (1) a ratio between the extension of compacted and noncompacted myocardium >2.3 measured on a longitudinal plane in the <>balanced TFE</> cine sequences *in diastole* (Fig. 3.6) and (2) a percentage of noncompacted left ventricular mass >20 % of the total mass (compacted+trabeculated) (Fig. 3.7). Even if the prevalence and significance of the intramyocardial fibrosis in this condition have not been determined, the delayed enhancement study is also of interest – as in dilated cardiomyopathy – for the purposes of prognostic stratification.

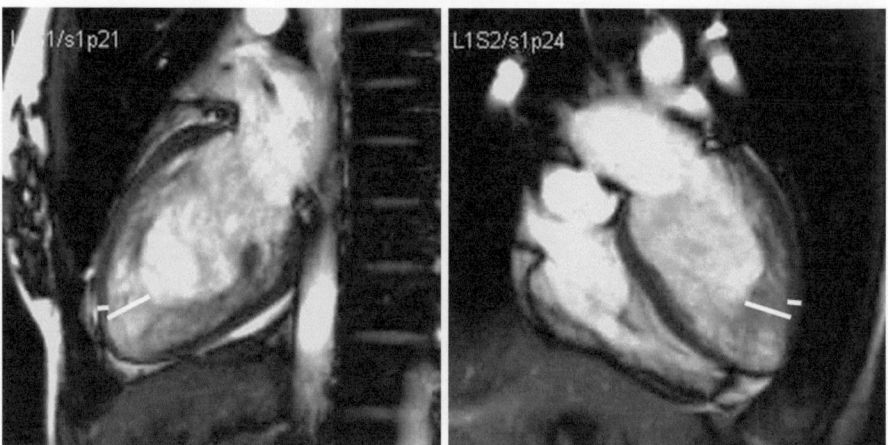

Fig. 3.6 Diastolic frames in two- (*left panel*) and four-chamber plane (*right panel*) from an SSFP cine sequence where measures of the extension of the noncompact layer and the compact myocardium are performed to calculate its ratio

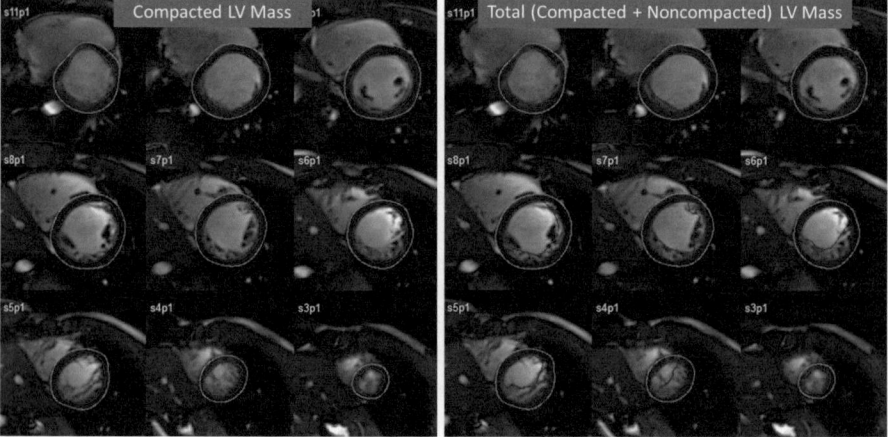

Fig. 3.7 Diastolic frames from short-axis SSFP cine sequences where the compact left ventricular mass is measured (*left panel*) and then the endocardial contour is adjusted to the limits of the noncompact layer (*right pa*nel) to estimate the "total" left ventricular mass. The difference between them related to the total mass will give the percentage of noncompact myocardium

3.5 Infiltrative and Restrictive Cardiomyopathies

The most frequent disease among infiltrative cardiomyopathies is cardiac amyloidosis, which consists of the extracellular deposition of insoluble fibrous protein material that interferes with the normal function of the organ in which it is located, in this case the myocardium. The myocardium is involved in more than

90 % of patients with systemic amyloidosis, although only in half of them is the process clinically relevant. When it is the case, the disease presents with signs and symptoms of heart failure mainly due to diastolic dysfunction. The CMR approach to cardiac amyloidosis follows the general protocol for cardiomyopathy detailed above. The cine sequences normally show diffuse, non-specific ventricular hypertrophy, normal or slightly reduced systolic function and biatrial dilation and hypertrophy, especially of the interatrial septum, where typically the membranous structures of the *fossa ovalis* are unaffected (see Fig. 3.8, arrow). These findings are not exclusive to amyloidosis, so delayed enhancement sequences are particularly important. In fact, diagnosis is frequently suspected in *Look-Locker* sequences when myocardial signal cannot be suppressed at any particular inversion time due to the disease's diffuse nature and the almost total absence of healthy myocardial tissue. Thus, the *IR TFE* delayed enhancement images show a pattern of diffuse enhancement that is frequently more intense in the subendocardial region (see Fig. 3.9), which is highly suggestive of cardiac amyloidosis.

In Fabry disease, a mutation of the gene that codifies the α-galactosidase enzyme causes a deficiency which leads to an abnormal storage of lipidic compounds in the lysosomes. CMR study shows left ventricle hypertrophy, which is also unspecific, and it is again the delayed enhancement study which guides the diagnosis, as in up to 50 % of cases a pattern of intramyocardial delayed enhancement may be observed, characteristically located in the basal inferolateral segment (see Fig. 3.10).

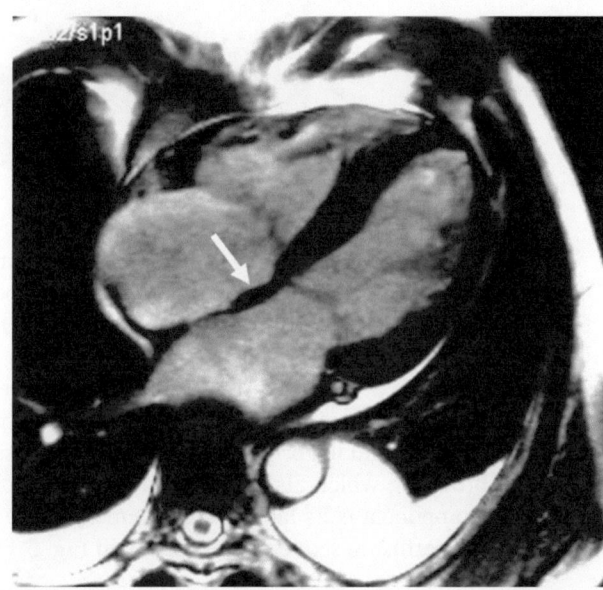

Fig. 3.8 Diastolic frame in four-chamber plane from an SSFP cine sequence in a patient with cardiac amyloidosis showing diffuse left ventricular hypertrophy and also increased thickness of the interatrial septum (*arrow*)

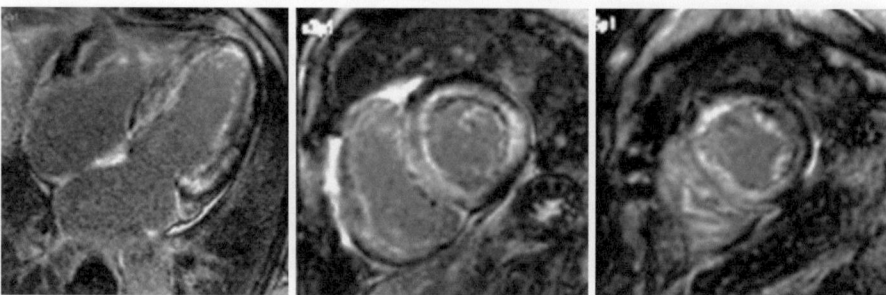

Fig. 3.9 IR TFE sequences showing delayed contrast enhancement with a diffuse pattern characteristic of cardiac amyloidosis

Fig. 3.10 IR TFE sequence in four-chamber view showing intramural delayed contrast enhancement located at the basal lateral region (*arrow*), typically seen in Fabry disease with cardiac involvement

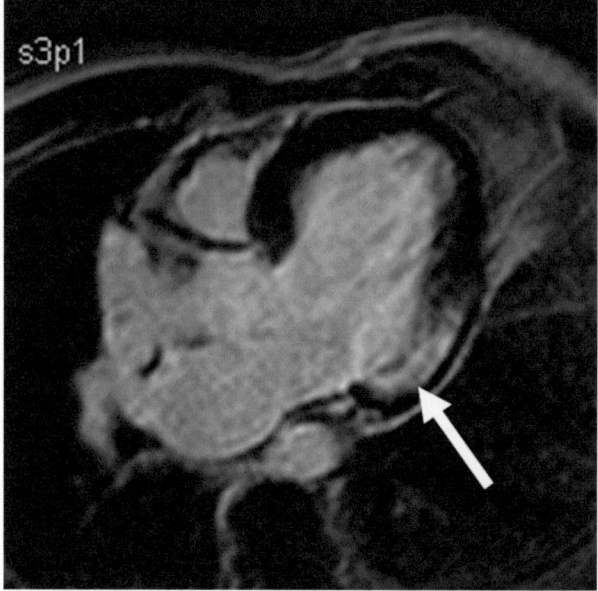

Endomyocardial fibrosis (EMF) is the most common restrictive cardiomyopathy. Of unknown origin, EMF consists of fibrotic tissue deposition in the endocardium of one or both ventricles and invariably leads to overt heart failure mainly due to diastolic heart failure. Delayed enhancement sequences are essential for diagnosis, as they may show a typical three-layered appearance (V sign) (see arrows in Fig. 3.11, left panel): the outer layer corresponds to normal myocardium, with low signal intensity; the middle, bright layer to the fibrous tissue; and the inner one to an overlying thrombus, which also has low intensity. A double check to identify this thrombotic component is its lack of enhancement in the first pass of contrast when studied with a perfusion sequence (see arrow in Fig. 3.11, right panel).

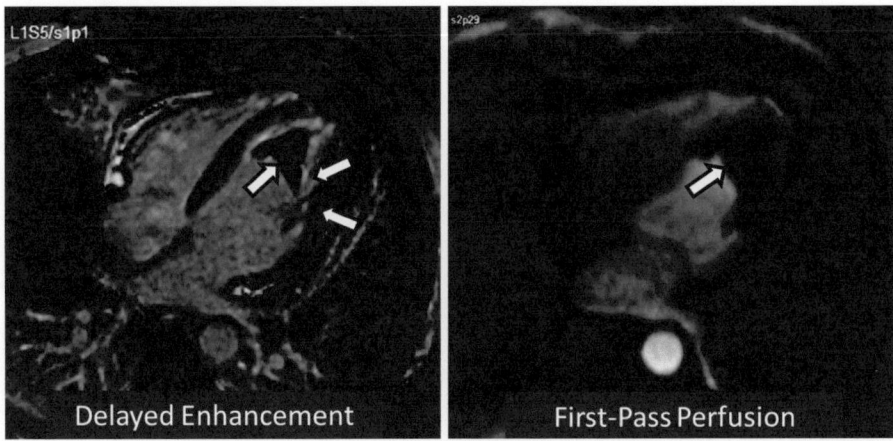

Fig. 3.11 IR TFE sequence (*left panel*) in a patient with endomyocardial fibrosis showing a characteristic three-layered V sign (*arrows*) consisting of the normal myocardium as an outward layer and enhanced medial layer corresponding to the endomyocardial fibrous tissue and an inner layer with dark signal intensity corresponding to overimposed thrombus. A first-pass perfusion sequence (*right panel*) in the same patient proves the non-vascularised nature of the thrombotic layer by its lack of enhancement (*arrow*)

3.6 Chagas Disease

Chagas disease is a chronic parasitic illness that is endemic in tropical areas of America and is caused by a *Trypanosoma cruzi* infection, which may affect the heart. Clinically overt cardiac involvement, which constitutes a true infective cardiomyopathy, presents in 30–40 % of all patients with the disease, and its most serious complication is extensive myocardial replacement by fibrotic scar, as shown in pathology studies. The CMR study protocol consists of the usual study of ventricular function and delayed enhancement. In the cine sequences, segmental contractile abnormalities may be observed, especially with wall thinning and aneurysms of the ventricular apical region (see Fig. 3.12, arrows), while delayed enhancement shows regional myocardial fibrosis, frequently transmural, although with a pattern of distribution that does not fit with specific territories of distribution of coronary arteries (Fig. 3.13, arrow).

3.7 Sarcoidosis

Sarcoidosis is an autoimmune, multisystemic, granulomatous disease of unknown origin, with symptomatic cardiac involvement in approximately 7 % of cases, although this may be present in subclinical form in up to 25 % of all patients with sarcoidosis. In this case, again, areas of bulging or dyskinesia of

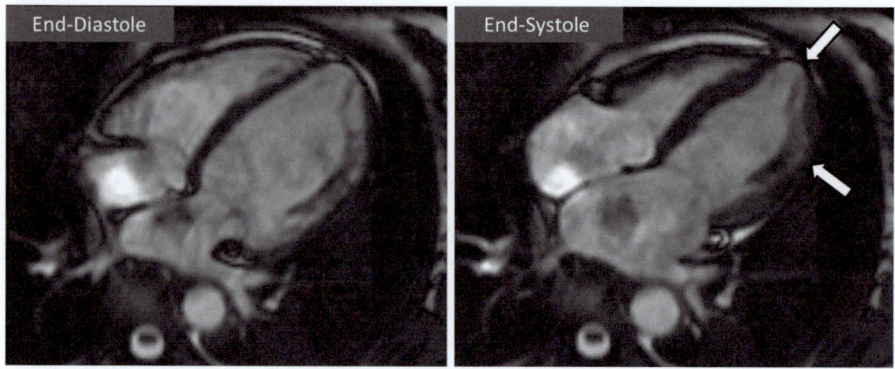

Fig. 3.12 Four-chamber SSFP images in end diastole (*left panel*) and end systole (*right panel*) showing areas of wall thinning and dyskinesia (*arrows*) in a patient with Chagas disease

Fig. 3.13 IR TFE sequence in four-chamber view from the same patient on Fig. 3.12 showing intramural delayed contrast enhancement indicating myocardial fibrosis located at the regions with wall thinning and contractile dysfunction

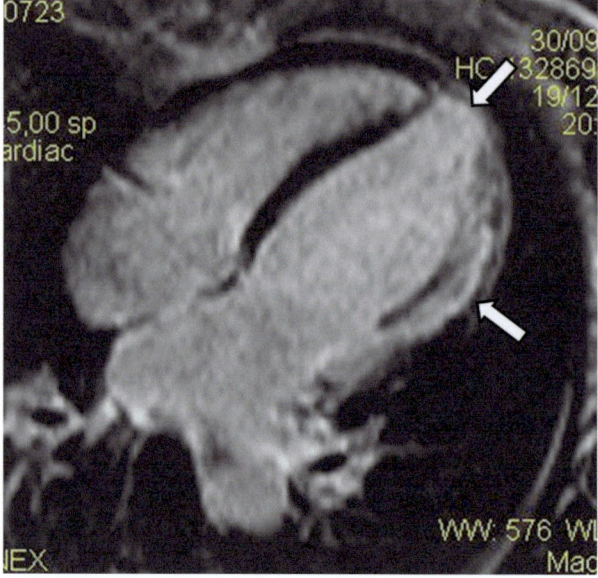

the left ventricle may appear (see Fig. 3.14, arrows in top and central panels) with a pattern of delayed enhancement that is frequently transmural and patchy and with a distribution that does not follow that of a particular coronary territory (see Fig. 3.14, arrows in bottom panel). The study protocol must include T2-weighted sequences to detect myocardial oedema as an expression of an active inflammatory process, which may regress as a response to treatment with corticoid agents.

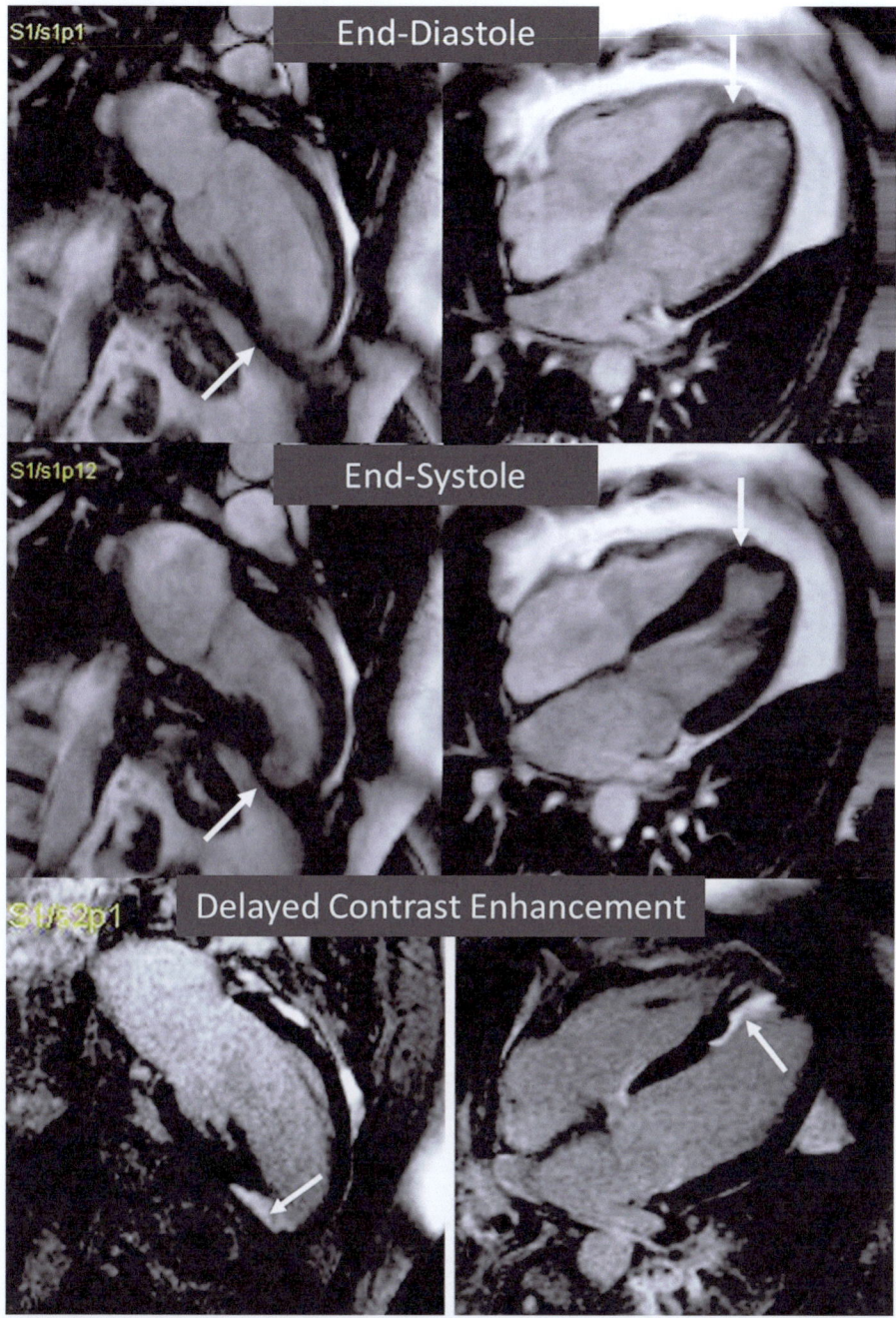

Fig. 3.14 SSFP images from two- and four-chamber cine sequences at end diastole (*upper panel*) and end systole (*middle panel*) showing areas of regional dyskinesia (*arrows*) in a patient with cardiac sarcoidosis, with correspondent myocardial scarring evidenced by delayed contrast enhancement in the IR TFE sequence (*arrows*, in *lower panel*)

3.8 Myocarditis

Myocarditis is a myocardial inflammatory process frequently of direct or immune-mediated viral origin, which presents in its acute phase with cellular oedema, necrosis and areas of inflammatory fibrosis. Myocarditis is a recognised cause of sudden death in young adults and must be considered in all patients with clinical signs of acute coronary syndrome, increased myocardial biomarkers and absence of angiographic coronary lesions.

When myocarditis is suspected, the basic CMR study protocol (function and delayed enhancement sequences) should be complemented by two additional types of sequences. First, a STIR series on longitudinal and transversal planes, which provides information on regional myocardial oedema (see Fig. 3.15, arrows), and, second, T1-weighted TSE sequences obtained before and immediately (1–2 min) after gadolinium contrast injection, which provides information on the presence of myocardial hyperaemia as an expression of regional vasodilation. As discussed in Chap. 1, oedema in STIR sequences is judged to be present when a ratio >2 is detected between the signal intensities of cardiac and skeletal muscles. The assessment of hyperaemia is made on the T1w TSE sequences by the so-called ratio of early myocardial enhancement (EMH), by which the increase in the myocardial (myoc) signal intensity (SI) is quantified after the administration of gadolinium (Gad), in relation to that observed in the skeletal muscle (ske) (see Fig. 3.16):

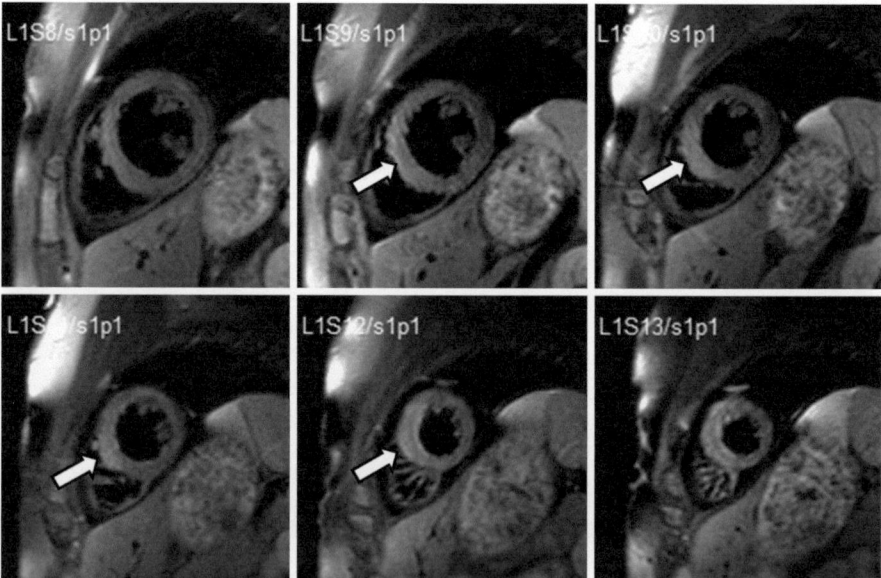

Fig. 3.15 Series of short-axis planes from a STIR sequence in a patient with acute myocarditis showing regional increased signal intensity (*arrows*) due to myocardial oedema

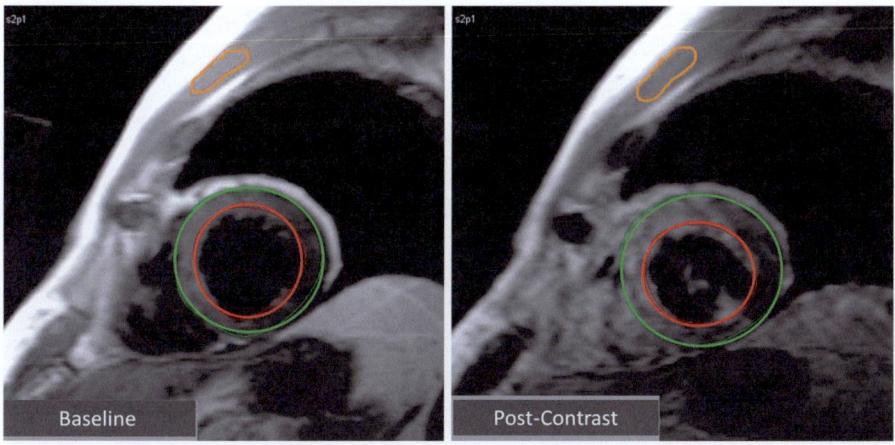

Fig. 3.16 T1w TSE sequences in short-axis view obtained before (*left panel*) and 1–2 min after contrast (*right panel*). Regions of interest have been located at the level of the entire left ventricular myocardium and at the skeletal muscle for the estimation of the ratio of early myocardial enhancement (see *text*)

$$\text{Ratio EMH} = \frac{\dfrac{SI_{myoc}\ post-Gad - SI_{myoc}\ pre-Gad}{SI_{myoc}\ pre-Gad}}{\dfrac{SI_{ske}\ post-Gad - SI_{ske}\ pre-Gad}{SI_{ske}\ pre-Gad}}$$

A value >4 of this ratio is indicative of myocardial hyperaemia.

In summary, the CMR study protocol for myocarditis follows the framework shown below.

Sequence	*Balanced TFE*	*Balanced TFE*	*Basal T1w TSE*	*STIR*
Information	2- and 4-chamber cine: function	Multiple short-axis cine: function	Hyperaemia	Myocardial edema

	Post-Gad T1w TSE	*Delayed IR TFE*
⟶	Hyperaemia	Necrosis and/or focal fibrosis

This protocol constitutes an important body of information for the diagnosis of myocarditis. It can be used to assess ventricular function both global and segmental, which, in the case of myocarditis, is usually impaired, although even when preserved the diagnosis cannot be excluded. It is also useful for the characterisation of myocardial tissue as it reveals oedema, hyperaemia and, as an essential element, areas of fibrosis. Such fibrosis presents with a non-ischaemic pattern and is characteristically located in the subepicardial region of the left ventricular free wall (arrows, in Fig. 3.17), though it may appear in patches elsewhere.

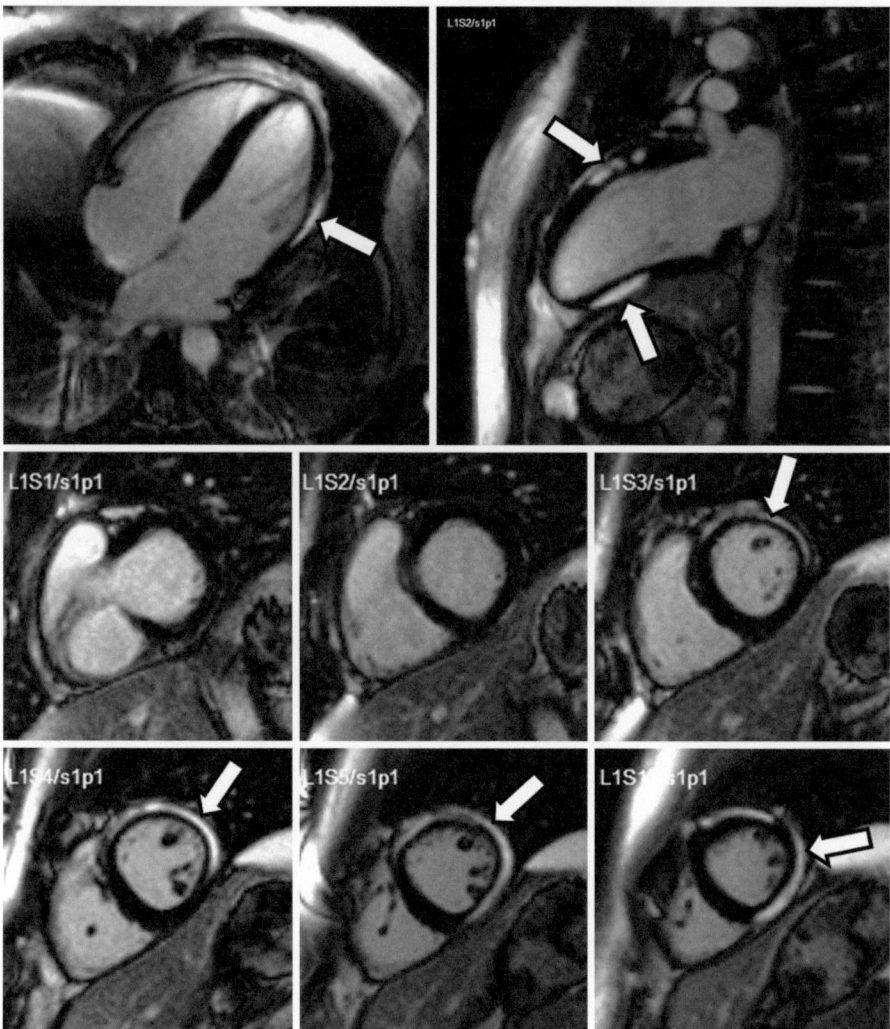

Fig. 3.17 IR TFE sequences in longitudinal (*upper row*) and short-axis planes (*middle* and *lower row*) in a case of acute myocarditis showing delayed enhancement with a typical distribution, involving the subepicardial aspect of the left ventricular free wall (*arrows*)

In practice, it is estimated that the diagnosis of myocarditis by CMR can be made when two of the following criteria are present:

1. Increased STIR signal intensity, which is indicative of myocardial oedema
2. Increased EMH ratio in T1w TSE, which is indicative of hyperaemia
3. Presence of focal delayed enhancement, with a non-ischaemic pattern, which is indicative of focal fibrosis

The additional observation of ventricular contractile dysfunction, global or regional, and/or pericardial effusion provides additional arguments to support the diagnosis.

3.9 Arrhythmogenic Right Ventricular Cardiomyopathy/Dysplasia (ARVC/D)

This genetic disease of the cardiac muscle presents with malign ventricular arrhythmias and, occasionally, with sudden death. Histopathologically, it is characterised by the replacement of the normal myocardium with fibroadipose tissue, which causes functional derangement and constitutes an arrhythmogenic substrate. It predominantly affects the right ventricle, but, in a proportion of patients, it also involves the left or both. Although CMR is an important diagnostic element, and in fact the suspicion of dysplasia is a frequent reason for study, the role of the technique is encompassed in a general diagnostic algorithm which includes other criteria besides imaging, such as family background, electrocardiographic abnormalities, presence and type of arrhythmias and even tissue analysis data by endomyocardial biopsy.

CMR findings that are currently considered in the diagnostic algorithm of ARVC/D include the presence of akinesia or focal dyskinesia of the right ventricular wall (see Fig. 3.18, arrows), along with dilation and/or systolic dysfunction of the chamber. Both segmental wall motion abnormality and global dysfunction of the right ventricle are required for diagnosis, although the specific data to consider in the algorithm for the diagnosis of ARVC/D is the end-diastolic volume of the right ventricle (EDVRV) and the right ventricular ejection

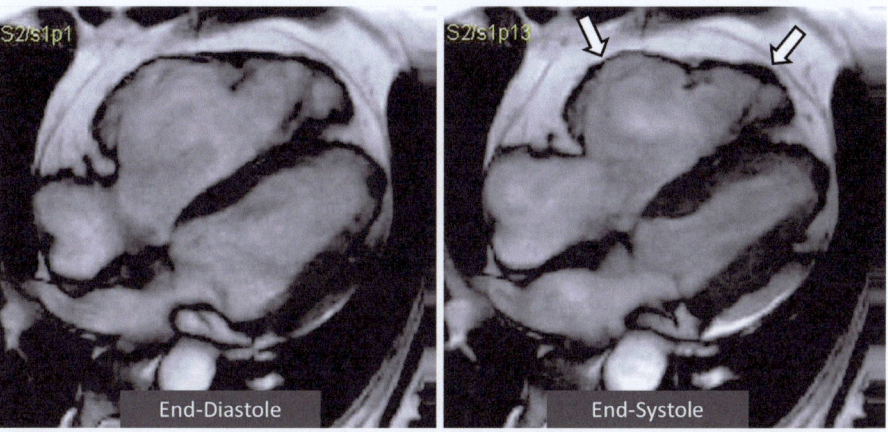

Fig. 3.18 Four-chamber SSFP images in end diastole (*left panel*) and end systole (*right panel*) showing significant right ventricular dilatation together with areas of right ventricular wall bulging and dyskinesia (*arrows*) in a patient with ARVC/D

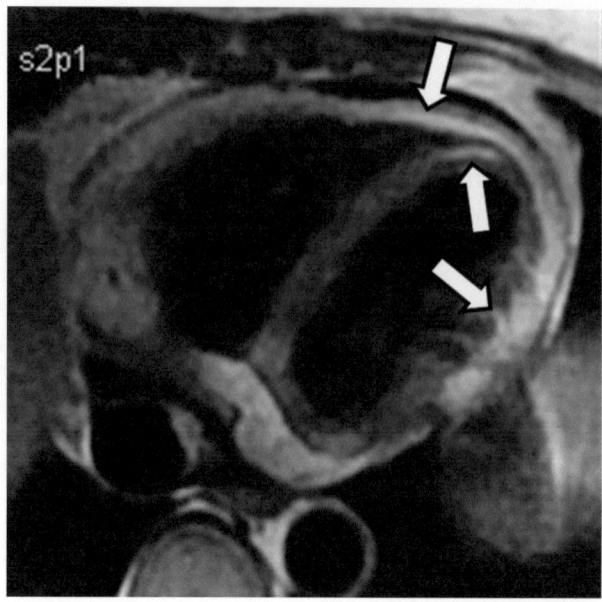

Fig. 3.19 T1w TSE sequence in transverse plane showing areas of high signal intensity indicating adipose infiltration of the right ventricular myocardium, the interventricular septum and, also, the subepicardial region of the left ventricular free wall (*arrows*) in a patient with ARVC/D with left ventricular involvement

fraction (RVEF). Thus, CMR can contribute to the diagnosis with the following criteria:

- Major criterion: right ventricular dysfunction + EDVRV (indexed) ≥ 110 ml/m^2 in men and ≥ 100 ml/m^2 in women and/or RVEF $\leq 40\%$
- Minor criterion: right ventricular dysfunction + EDVRV (indexed) ≥ 100 ml/m^2 and <110 ml/m^2 in men and ≥ 90 ml/m^2 and <100 ml/m^2 in women and/or RVEF $>40\%$ and $\leq 45\%$

Given that diagnostic certainty in ARVC/D requires the presence of at least two major criteria (or one major and two minor; or four minor), it is deduced that the positive findings of a CMR study such as the ones mentioned do not allow, in the absence of other criteria, more than the diagnosis of "possible" ARVC/D.

The histopathological basis of the disease is the replacement of the right ventricular myocardium with fibroadipose tissue, which may be apparent in CMR using T1w TSE and delayed enhancement sequences, which may, respectively, show the presence of fatty tissue in the right and/or left ventricular wall (arrows, in Fig. 3.19) or focal myocardial fibrosis (arrow, in Fig. 3.20). Although part of a comprehensive CMR study of ARVC/D, these findings have not been included as diagnostic criteria because

Fig. 3.20 IR TFE sequence in short-axis plane showing delayed enhancement of the right ventricular wall (*arrow*) in a patient with ARVC/D

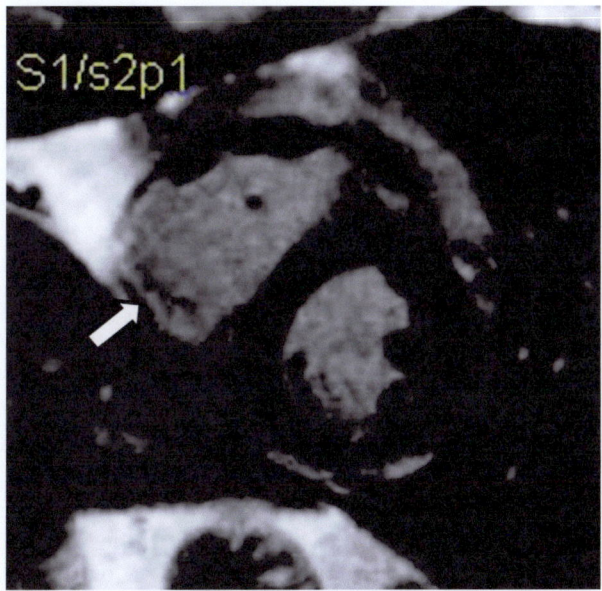

Fig. 3.21 T1w TSE sequence in transverse plane showing an area of high signal intensity due to adipose tissue (*arrow*) in the apical region of the right ventricular wall in an otherwise normal subject

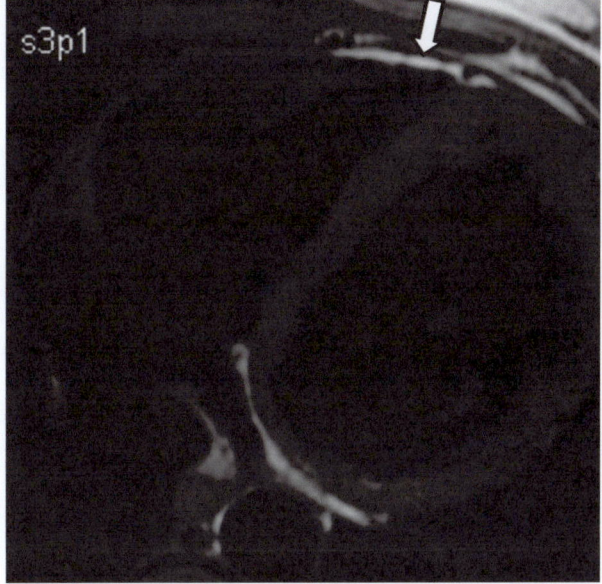

of frequent uncertainty in their assessment, given the reduced thickness of the right ventricular wall and the presence of wall fat in otherwise normal individuals (see Fig. 3.21, arrow).

In summary, the complete CMR study protocol for ARVC/D includes the following steps:

Sequence	Balanced TFE	Balanced TFE	Balanced TFE	Balanced TFE
Information	2- and 4-chamber cine: function	Multiple short-axis cine: function	2-Chamber of the right ventricle: function	Sagittal slices of the right ventricular outflow tract: function

	Axial T1w TSE	Delayed IR TFE
⟶	Characterisation of the right ventricular wall	Necrosis and/or focal fibrosis

Given that the functional assessment of the right ventricle is determinant in the diagnostic algorithm of this condition, the study protocol should be fundamentally focussed on an exhaustive evaluation of its global and segmental contractility. For this reason, in addition to the standard protocol of the function study (see Chap. 1, Figs. 1.3, 1.4, 1.5, 1.6 and 1.7), cine sequences will be obtained in a vertical longitudinal plane of the right ventricle (two chambers of the inflow tract) and sagittal planes oriented on the outflow chamber of the right ventricle, to assess motion in all regions of what is known as the "dysplasia triangle": inflow chamber, infundibulum or outflow tract and apex of the right ventricle.

As mentioned above, information on fatty or fibrous tissue in the right ventricular wall is not considered in the strict diagnostic algorithm of the disease, although it is recommended to investigate their presence, as they may turn out to be key elements supporting the diagnosis of ARVC/D in cases of borderline results of the conventional data.

3.10 Cardiomyopathy due to Iron Overload

Abnormal myocardial iron deposits may appear in hereditary haemochromatosis and in chronic anaemias that require continuous transfusions, such as *thalassemia major*. Their detection is important, as cardiomyopathy due to iron deposition may present with heart failure if not appropriately treated earlier. There are no distinctive morphological or functional traits of cardiac iron overload detectable by CMR, particularly at early stages. Importantly, however, the technique allows for an estimate of the concentration of myocardial iron by measuring the $T2^*$ relaxation time, a parameter that is related to the level of inhomogeneity of the tissue being studied, which is altered by the presence of iron, that, in turn, notably shortens the $T2^*$ value. A myocardial $T2^* < 20$ ms (when studied with 1.5 T systems) means a significant iron overload, which is

3 CMR Study Protocol of Cardiomyopathies

associated with cardiac insufficiency. To measure the T2* value of the myocardium, a TSE sequence is used which acquires up to eight images on a single plane at increasing echo times (TE). A region of interest (ROI) is traced in the interventricular septum (in the same position in all the images) to calculate the signal intensity (SI) in each image, corresponding to the various ETs (see Fig. 3.22). The data can be put into a graph, from which, by computing the SI and TE, the T2* curve is obtained, the numerical value of which is given by an exponential logarithm calculation (see Fig. 3.23).

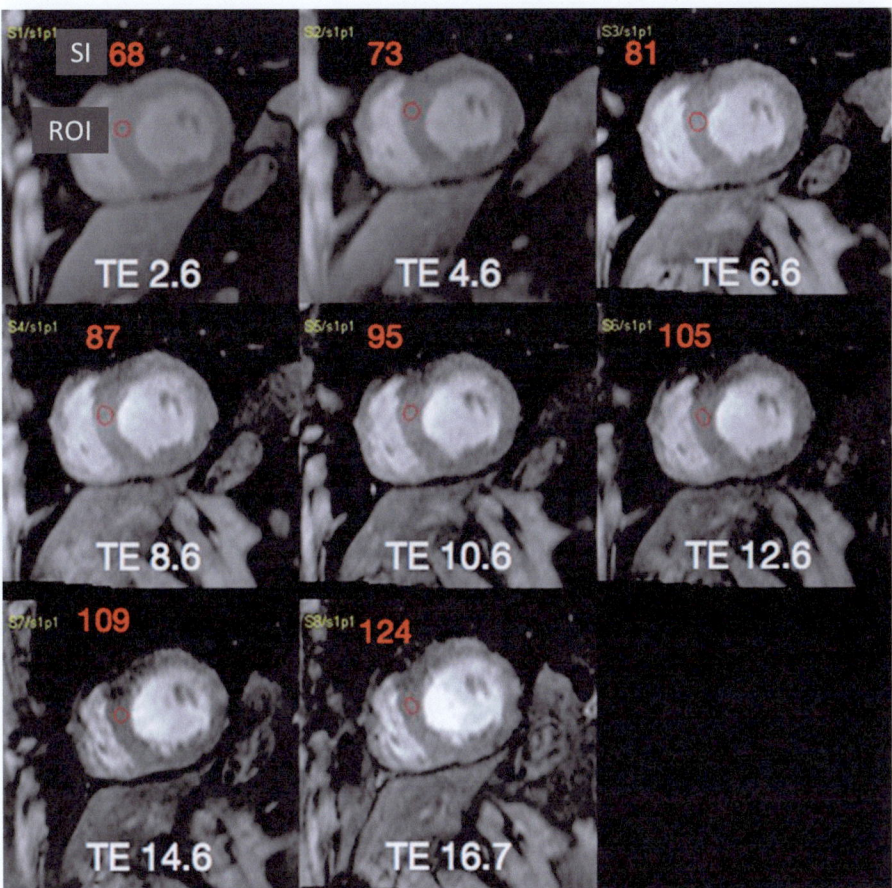

Fig. 3.22 TSE sequence on a short-axis plane with progressively increased echo time (*TE*) where signal intensity (*SI*) is measured at a region of interest (*ROI*) in each image to estimate the myocardial T2* value

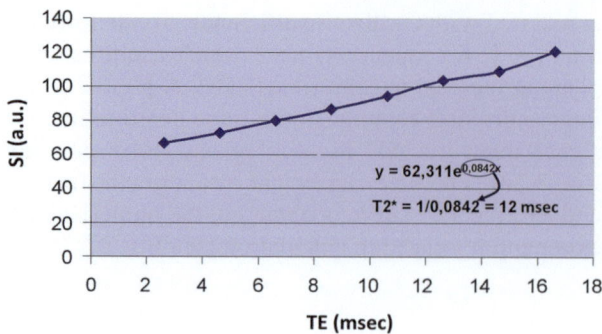

Fig. 3.23 Graphics showing the logarithmical curve obtained from the myocardial signal intensity and the corresponding TE as obtained in Fig. 3.22 and the equation for calculation of the myocardial T2* value

Recommended Bibliography

1. Almehmadi F, Joncas SX, Nevis I, Zahrani M, Bokhari M, Stirrat J et al (2014) Prevalence of myocardial fibrosis patterns in patients with systolic dysfunction. Prognostic significance for the prediction of sudden cardiac arrest or appropriate implantable cardiac defibrillator therapy. Circ Cardiovasc Imaging 7:593–600
2. Chan RH, Maron BJ, Olivotto I (2014) Prognostic value of quantitative contrast-enhanced cardiovascular magnetic resonance for the evaluation of sudden death risk in patients with hypertrophic cardiomyopathy. Circulation 130:484–495
3. Dungu JN, Valencia O, Pinney JH, Gibbs SDJ, Rowczenio D, Gilbertson JA et al (2014) CMR-based differentiation of AL and ATTR Cardiac Amyloidosis. J Am Coll Cardiol Img 7:133–142
4. Friedrich MG, Sechtem U, Schulz-Menger J, Holmvang G, Alakija P, Cooper LT et al (2009) Cardiovascular magnetic resonance in myocarditis: a JACC white paper. J Am Coll Cardiol 53:1475–1487
5. Friedrich MG, Marcotte F (2013) Cardiac magnetic resonance assessment of myocarditis. Circ Cardiovasc Imaging 6:833–839
6. Jacquier A, Thuny F, Jop B, Giorgi R, Cohen F, Gaubert JY et al (2010) Measurement of trabeculated left ventricular mass using cardiac magnetic resonance imaging in the diagnosis of left ventricular non-compaction. Eur Heart J 31:1098–1104
7. Karamitsos TD, Francis JM, Myerson S, Selvanayagam JB, Neubauer S (2009) The role of cardiovascular magnetic resonance imaging in heart failure. J Am Coll Cardiol 54:1407–1424
8. Marcus FI, McKenna WJ, Sherrill D, Basso C, Bauce B, Bluemke DA et al (2010) Diagnosis of arrhythmogenic right ventricular cardiomyopathy/dysplasia. Proposed modifications of the task force criteria. Circulation 121:1533–1541
9. Maron MS (2012) Clinical utility of cardiovascular magnetic resonance in hypertrophic cardiomyopathy. J Cardiovasc Magn Reson 14:13
10. Patel MR, Cawley PJ, Heitner JF, Kelm I, Parker MA, Jaroudi WA et al (2009) Detection of myocardial damage in patients with sarcoidosis. Circulation 120:1969–1977
11. Rochitte CE, Oliveira PF, Andrade JM, Ianni BM, Parga JR, Avila LF et al (2005) Myocardial delayed enhancement by magnetic resonance imaging in patients with Chagas' disease: a marker of disease severity. J Am Coll Cardiol 46:1553–1558
12. Salemi VMC, Rochitte CE, Shiozaki AA, Andrade JM, Parga JR, de Avila LF et al (2011) Late gadolinium enhancement magnetic resonance imaging in the diagnosis and prognosis of endomyocardial fibrosis patients. Circ Cardiovasc Imaging 4:304–311

13. Schumm J, Greulich S, Wagner A, Grün S, Ong P, Bentz K et al (2014) Cardiovascular magnetic resonance risk stratification in patients with clinically suspected myocarditis. J Cardiovasc Magn Reson 16:14
14. Smith GC, Carpenter JP, He T, Alam MH, Firmin DN, Pennell DJ (2011) Value of black blood T2* cardiovascular magnetic resonance. J Cardiovasc Magn Reson 13:21
15. te Riele A, Tandri H, Bluemke D (2014) Arrhythmogenic right ventricular cardiomyopathy (ARVC): cardiovascular magnetic resonance update. J Cardiovasc Magn Reson 16:50

CMR Study Protocol of Pericardial Diseases

Francesc Carreras

4.1 Introduction

Imaging techniques have facilitated the diagnosis of pericardial diseases. Echocardiography continues to be the technique of choice, but is frequently limited by images that are difficult to interpret or by discrepancies with other clinical findings. The contribution of cardiovascular magnetic resonance (CMR) is therefore important, its main advantages being the wide field of vision it provides, its capacity for tissue characterisation and its possible use for a dynamic study of the effects of pericardial abnormalities on the normal motion of the heart chambers. It should be mentioned that computed tomography also has a role in the study of pericardial diseases, particularly the detection of pericardial calcifications, a finding that is occasionally essential in the diagnosis of pericardial constriction and for which echocardiography and CMR have limited capacity.

4.2 Sequence Protocol for the Study of Pericardial Diseases

1. *Localiser sequences* (see Chap. 1, Fig. 1.2): these are useful for a first look at the dimensions of the inferior vena cava and the presence of pericardial effusion and, also, of pleural effusion and/or ascites as extracardiac findings potentially related to the pericardial process.
2. *Axial multi-slice with T1w TSE sequences* (see Chap. 1, Fig. 1.13): allow the estimation of the thickness and the morphological features of the pericardium, the detection of the presence of effusion and the assessment of the intensity of its signal, which is useful for identifying the character of the fluid.

F. Carreras, MD, PhD
Cardiac Imaging Unit, Cardiology Department, Hospital de la Santa Creu i Sant Pau,
Universitat Autònoma de Barcelona, Barcelona, Spain
e-mail: fcarreras@santpau.cat

3. *Short-axis multi-slice with STIR sequences* (see Chap. 1, Fig. 1.1b): used for the detection of pericardial/myocardial oedema.
4. *Longitudinal and short-axis balanced-TFE cines* (see Chap. 1, Figs. 1.3–1.7): used to detect pericardial effusion, to study its dynamics and to analyse ventricular function, particularly the pattern of septal motion.
5. *Balanced FFE short-axis cine in real time with forced respiration*: used for the analysis of ventricular interdependence (pattern of septal motion) and the morphological variations of the ventricular chambers during free breathing.
6. *Sequence of myocardial tagging on short-axis planes* (see Chap. 1, Fig. 1.1f): useful for analysing myocardial rotation and torsion and their impairment in case of adherence to the pericardial layers.
7. *Inversion recovery turbo field echo (IR-TFE) sequences on axial, longitudinal and short-axis planes* (see Chap. 1, Fig. 1.17): acquired 10 min after the injection of gadolinium at a dose of 0.2 mmol/kg, it is used for the detection of delayed enhancement in the pericardium/myocardium.

4.3 Morphological Study of the Pericardium

The morphological study of the pericardium is based on *T1w-TSE* and *balanced-TFE* sequences. In *T1w-TSE* sequences, the normal pericardium is shown with a hypointense, curvilinear and homogeneous signal which is surrounded by high-intensity signals from the epicardial and paracardiac fat (see Fig. 4.1, arrows). The pericardial signal includes its two components – visceral and parietal – and the small amount of physiological pericardial fluid, which corresponds to ultrafiltrated plasma (10–50 ml). The maximal thickness of the normal pericardium measured by CMR is 2–2.5 mm, with a value >4 mm being considered definitively abnormal. However, at the level of the superior pericardial recesses of the large vessels, the pericardium may show a greater thickness even in normal conditions if the patient is lying down. The pericardial signal is not necessarily visualised throughout its whole extension, as this depends on the presence of fatty tissue at its borders; due to the frequent lack of it at the posterior aspect of the heart, the pericardium may appear to be absent at this

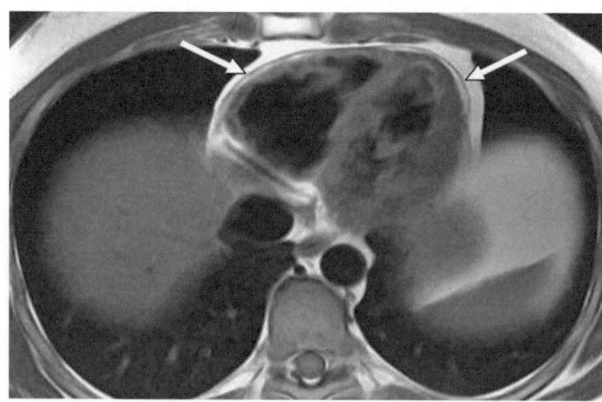

Fig. 4.1 T1w-TSE sequence in transverse plane showing the signal corresponding to the pericardium (*arrows*)

Fig. 4.2 T1w-TSE sequence in coronal plane in a case of congenital absence of the pericardium showing displacement of cardiac chambers to the left hemithorax (*horizontal arrow*) and normal central position of extrapericardial structures (*vertical arrow*)

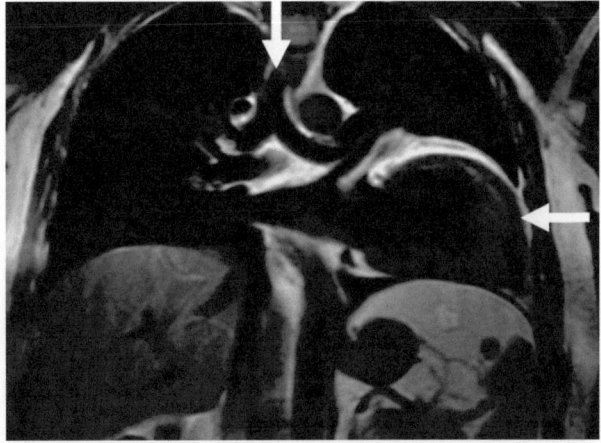

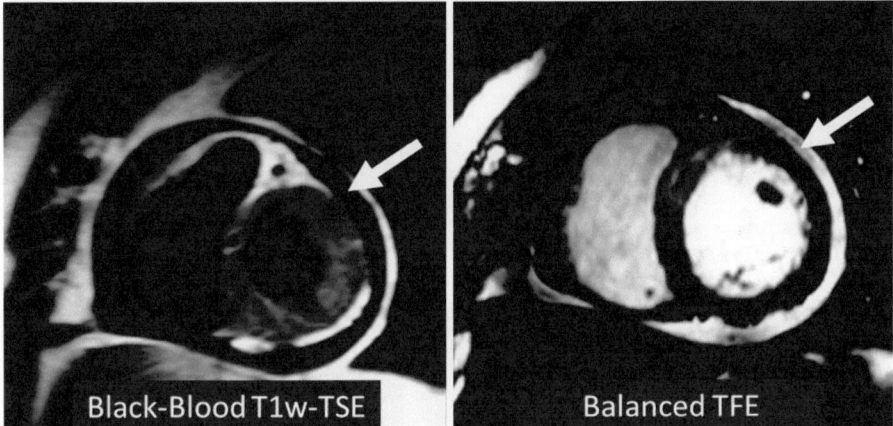

Fig. 4.3 T1w-TSE sequence in short-axis plane (*left panel*) and SSFP image (*right panel*) at the same level in a case of pericardial effusion (*arrows*)

level. Thus, a congenital absence of the pericardium, whether partial or total, cannot be confirmed by the simple absence of pericardial signal. Rather, in this case there are indirect signs which must be searched for, such as the herniation or abnormal displacement of the cardiac cavities towards the left hemithorax (see Fig. 4.2, horizontal arrow), while the extrapericardial mediastinal structures, such as the trachea, remain in their normal, central position (see Fig. 4.2, vertical arrow).

Both the increase in the pericardial space >4 mm and the loss of the regular contour of the pericardial signal, with areas of irregular thickening, indicate the presence of an abnormal pericardial process. In *T1w-TSE* sequences, increased pericardial thickness with low intensity of signal may correspond either to an effusion (see Fig. 4.3, arrow in the left panel) or to an abnormal thickening of the pericardial layers without any significant amount of fluid (see Fig. 4.4, arrow in the left panel). *Balanced-TFE* cine sequences on the same orientation should be analysed, in which high signal intensity will be shown in the case of an effusion (see Fig. 4.3,

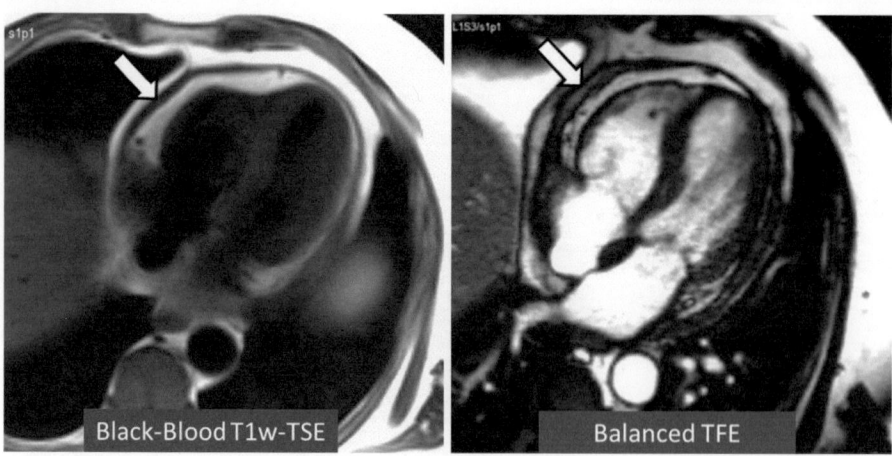

Fig. 4.4 T1w-TSE sequence in four-chamber plane (*left panel*) and SSFP image (*right panel*) at the same level in a case of thickened pericardium without effusion (*arrows*)

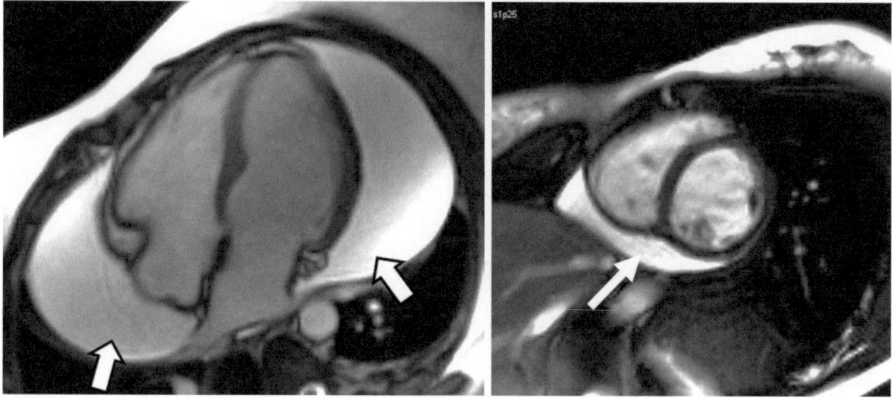

Fig. 4.5 SSFP images from two chambers and short-axis cine sequences in a case of large massive pericardial effusion (*arrows, left panel*) and in a moderate effusion located at the inferior pericardial space (*arrow, right panel*)

arrow in the right panel) and low signal if there is pericardial thickening without effusion (see Fig. 4.4, right panel). The latter finding constitutes a key element for the diagnosis of pericardial constriction by CMR.

The visualisation of cine sequences is also useful. In the case of an effusion, changes occur in the shape of the pericardial space throughout the cardiac cycle due to redistribution of fluid, which are not present in case of increased pericardial space without effusion. In general, pericardial effusion is diffuse, although it may appear as predominantly located, by the effect of gravity, in the lower regions of the pericardial space (see arrows in Fig. 4.5, left panel). Strictly localised effusions, however, may also exist (see Fig. 4.5, arrow on the right panel).

Fig. 4.6 T1w-TSE sequence in transverse plane showing the dark signal of a pericardial effusion (*black arrow*) and the bright signal produced by adipose epicardial tissue (*white arrow*)

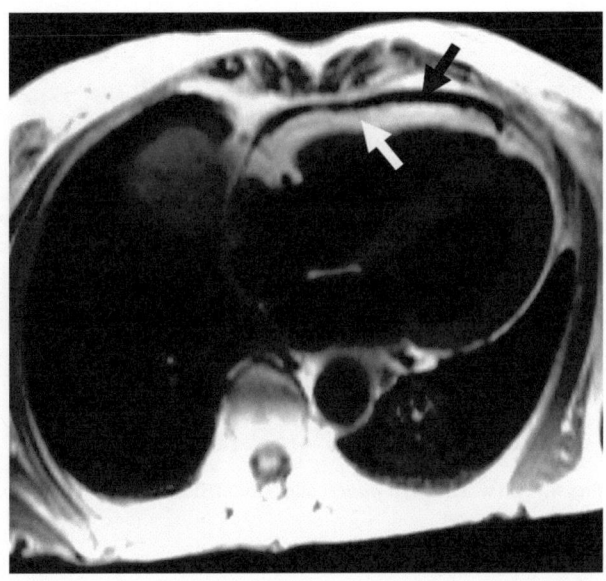

4.4 Study of Tissue Characterisation in Pericardial Pathology

The ability to distinguish the tissue composition of different structures according to their signal intensity in particular CMR sequences is an aspect of interest in the study of pericardial pathology. First of all, for the recognition of pericardial effusion itself, which is occasionally unclear by echocardiography (e.g.: apparently increased anterior pericardial space, which can be due to, either, effusion, or to profuse epicardial adipose tissue). In this case, *T1w-TSE-T1* sequences show a clear difference between the high intensity of the signal in the case of fatty tissue (see Fig. 4.6, white arrow) and the low signal of a true effusion (see Fig. 4.6, black arrow).

The nature of the fluid in a pericardial effusion will induce different signal intensities depending on the type of sequence applied: a combined analysis can allow its character to be assessed. The following table is a guide:

Pericardial contents	T1w-TSE	T2w-TSE	Balanced-TFE
Transudate	Low	High	High
Exudate	Medium	Medium	High
Haemorrhage	High	High	High
Air	Low	Low	Low

Similarly, when a pericardial cyst is suspected, the combined use of sequences is useful for its confirmation, showing low signal intensity in *T1w-TSE* (see Fig. 4.7,

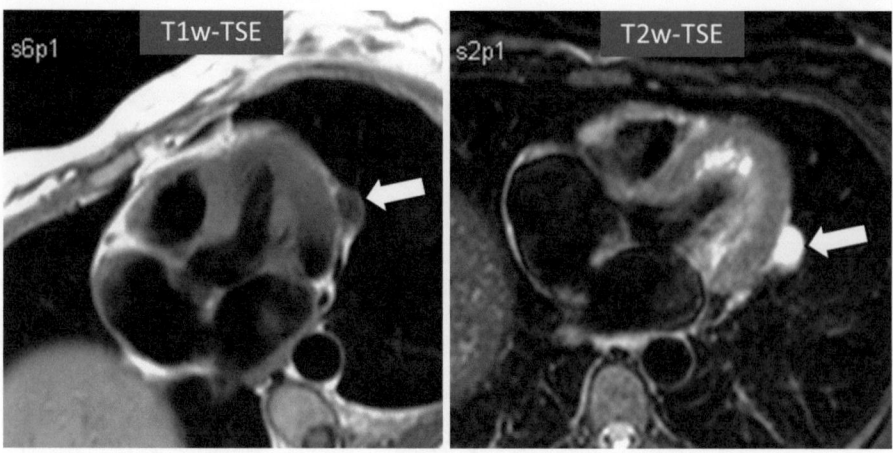

Fig. 4.7 T1w-TSE (*left panel*) and T2w-TSE sequence (*right panel*) images in a case of pericardial cyst (*arrows*)

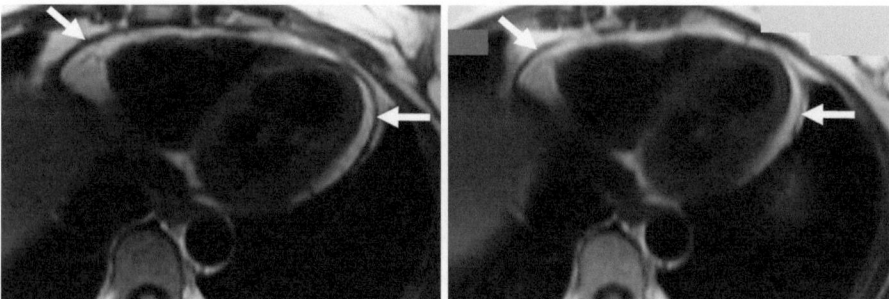

Fig. 4.8 T1w-TSE sequence in transverse plane in the same patient obtained at the acute phase of pericarditis (*left panel*) and after resolution (*right panel*), showing reduction of pericardial thickness (*arrows*)

arrow in the left panel) and very high in *T2w-TSE* (see Fig. 4.7, arrow in the right panel), allowing the liquid content to be confirmed, which is diagnostic of a pericardial cyst.

The process of pericardial inflammation, whether acute or chronically active, leads to an increase in pericardial thickness detectable in *T1w-TSE* sequences (see Fig. 4.8, arrows in the left panel), which may recede in follow-up studies in the case of regression of an acute pericarditis (see Fig. 4.8, arrows in the right-hand panel). On the other hand, the inflammatory process of the pericardium will cause delayed contrast enhancement in IR-TFE sequences. The pericardium appears then with a hyperintense signal (see Fig. 4.9, arrows), which is characteristic of acute pericarditis, or chronic with a persistent inflammatory component.

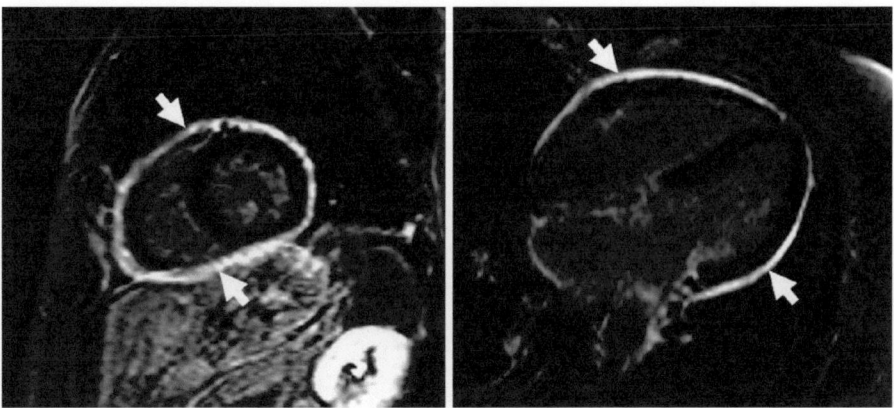

Fig. 4.9 IR-TFE sequences in short- and long-axis planes showing delayed enhancement of the pericardium (*arrows*) in a case of acute pericarditis

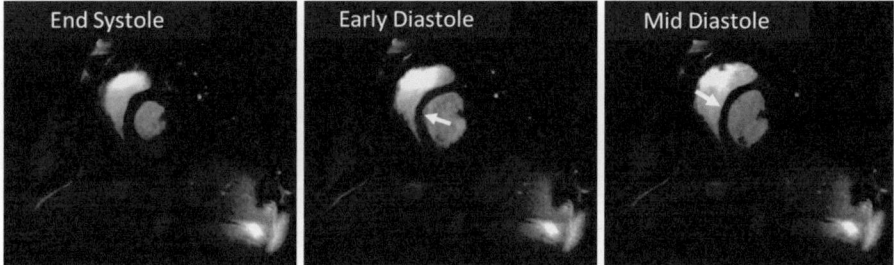

Fig. 4.10 Frames from a short-axis SSFP cine sequence in a case of constrictive pericarditis showing an abrupt early diastolic displacement of the interventricular septum towards the right ventricle (*arrow*, in *central panel*) which recovers its normal position at mid-diastole (*arrow*, in *right panel*)

4.5 Functional Study of Pericardial Diseases

The analysis of cardiac function through *balanced-TFE* cine sequences allows the detection of signs of impaired ventricular filling due to pericardial effusion or constriction. One of these signs is a rebound of the interventricular septum in early diastole (arrows, in Fig. 4.10) as an expression of the sudden constraint found by the filling ventricles. The behaviour of the interventricular septum during the respiratory cycle is also altered in these cases and requires a study with cine sequences in real time during forced free breathing. This allows, in cases of constriction, the detection of a flattening of the interventricular septum towards the left ventricle during inhalation (arrow in Fig. 4.11, left panel) which normalises upon exhalation (Fig. 4.11, right panel).

Finally, in pericardial constriction, there is a process of adherence to the pericardial layers which may involve the epicardial surface of the heart, preventing the

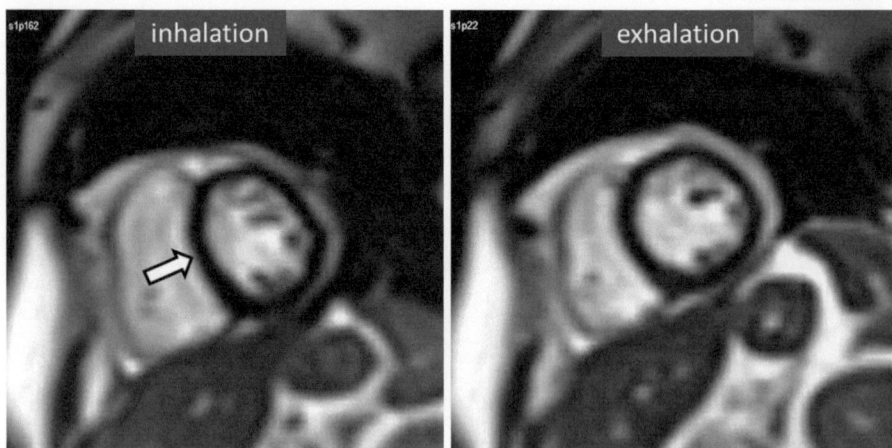

Fig. 4.11 Frames from a real-time cine sequence showing a flattening of the interventricular septum during inhalation (*arrow, left panel*) which normalises at exhalation

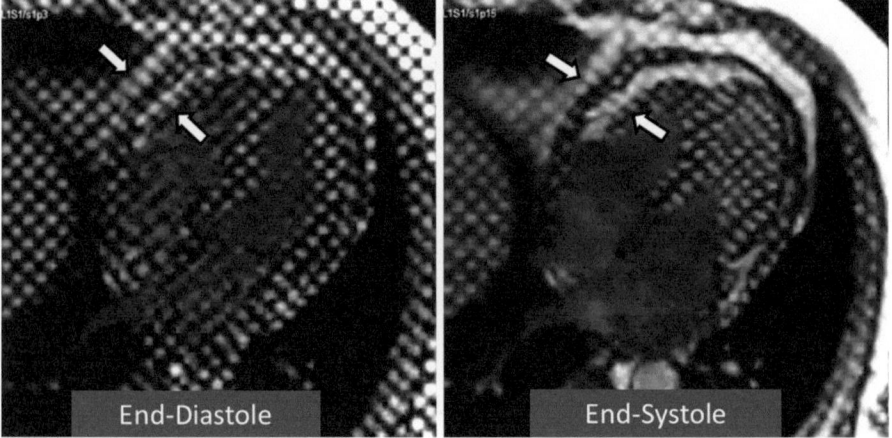

Fig. 4.12 Frames from a tagging cine sequence in four-chamber view showing continuity of presaturation lines from diastole to systole (*arrows*) due to epicardial-to-pericardial adherence in a case of constriction

normal radial and longitudinal slippage motion of the ventricles. This may be studied by tagging cine sequences, where presaturation lines from the pericardial space and the underlying myocardium remain unbroken throughout the cardiac cycle (see arrows in Figs. 4.4, 4.5, 4.6, 4.7, 4.8, 4.9, 4.10, 4.11, and 4.12), indicating the adherence of the pericardium to the epicardium.

Recommended Bibliography

1. Bogaert J, Francote M (2009) Cardiovascular magnetic resonance in pericardial diseases. J Cardiovasc Magn Reson 11:14
2. Cosyns B, Plein S, Nihoyanopoulos P, Smiseth O, Achenbach S, Andrade MJ et al (2015) European Association of Cardiovascular Imaging (EACVI) position paper: multimodality imaging in pericardial disease. Eur Heart J Cardiovasc Imaging 16:12–31
3. Rajiah P, Cardiac MRI (2011) Part 2. Pericardial diseases. Am J Roentgenol 197:W621

CMR Study Protocol of Cardiac Masses and Tumours

5

Francesc Carreras and Alberto Hidalgo

5.1 Introduction

In daily practice, the use of cardiovascular magnetic resonance (CRM) to examine a cardiac or paracardiac mass will normally be prompted by its detection in a prior echocardiographic study. From the epidemiological point of view, it must be borne in mind that the most frequently encountered intracardiac mass is an intracavitary thrombus; cardiac and pericardial tumours are rare and the majority of them are myxomas – the most common benign tumour (75 % of the total) – sarcomas, the most commonly found malign tumours, are much less common (15 %). In general, paracardiac masses are a more frequent cause for a CMR study than intracardiac ones, and their clinical significance depends on the potential for compression or displacement of the cardiac chambers.

For the study of a mass, CMR is preferred to echocardiography for several reasons: larger field of view, lack of interference from other structures, higher image resolution and the possibility of tissue characterisation through the use of different study sequences. Images acquired by CMR allow the identification of myocardium, pericardium, pericardial fat, the coronary arteries, the large vessels and the rest of the thoracic structures. In contrast to echocardiography, the wide field of view allows the unlimited observation of the extension of the mass and its anatomical relations with the pulmonary and mediastinal structures. The information obtained is of interest for a first approach to the aetiology of a mass and is especially useful for planning surgical removal of the mass, if necessary.

F. Carreras, MD, PhD (✉)
Cardiac Imaging Unit, Cardiology Department, Hospital de la Santa Creu i Sant Pau,
Universitat Autònoma de Barcelona, Barcelona, Spain
e-mail: fcarreras@santpau.cat

A. Hidalgo, MD, PhD
Cardiac Imaging Unit, Radiology Department, Hospital de la Santa Creu i Sant Pau,
Universitat Autònoma de Barcelona, Barcelona, Spain

5.2 Protocol of Recommended Sequences and Image Analysis

In practice, the study of a cardiac mass of unclear aetiology should be performed systematically. We recommend the application of the following sequences (detailed in Chap. 1):

Axial T1w-TSE	Axial T2w TSE+STIR	Multislice *balanced-FFE*	First-pass perfusion	Post-contrast Axial T1w-TSE	Delayed IR-TFE

The aim of this study is to accurately describe the features of the mass as a first step for a diagnostic approach of its nature (see Table 5.1). It is useful to evaluate the size and shape of the mass, its anatomical relationships and its impact on the function of the heart. Of particular importance is the study of its borders which, when ill-defined and infiltrative of neighbouring structures, suggest a fast growth process that is probably malign, which is frequently accompanied by pericardial or pleural effusion. Cine sequences are especially useful for analysing the motion pattern of the mass and its interaction with other structures. Likewise, through the characteristics of the signal in the different sequences and the changes observed with the administration of contrast, we can attempt a tissue characterisation of the mass.

With this data, it is our aim to disclose the origin of the mass or, at least, to distinguish between those of benign and malign character (see Table 5.2) for which the location of

Table 5.1 Aspects to be specified in the study of cardiac masses by CMR

	Morphology	Localization
		Shape
		Borders
		Motion
	Characterisation	Signal intensity
		Homogeneity/heterogeneity
		Vascularization
		Tissue fibrosis
	Associated findings	Pericardial/Pleural effusion
		Extracardiac extension

Table 5.2 Cardiac tumours

Primary		Secondary		
Benign	Malign	Direct extension	Venous extension	Metastatic extension
Myxoma Fibroma Lipoma Fibroelastoma Rhabdomyoma Haemangioma	Sarcoma mesothelioma Lymphoma	Lung Breast Oesophagus Mediastinum	Renal Suprarenal Liver Thyroid Lung Uterus	Melanoma, leukaemia, lymphoma Genital Urinary gastrointestinal

5 CMR Study Protocol of Cardiac Masses and Tumours

Table 5.3 Probable type of tumour according to location

Localization	Probable diagnosis	Others
Left atrium (intracavitary)	Myxoma	Sarcoma, metastasis, haemangioma, thrombus
Left atrium (intramural)	Sarcoma	Lymphoma, metastasis
Right atrium (intracavitary)	Myxoma	Thrombus, metastasis, haemangioma
Right atrium (intramural)	Angiosarcoma	Lipomatous hypertrophy
Left ventricle (intracavitary)	Uncertain	Sarcoma, lipoma, haemangioma, thrombus
Left ventricle (intramural)	Uncertain	Sarcoma, lipoma, haemangioma
Pericardium	Metastasis	Mesothelioma, lymphoma, sarcoma, haemangioma
Valvular	Papillary fibroelastoma	Myxoma

Table 5.4 Differential diagnosis of tumours by CMR

In favour of benignity	In favour of malignity
Left chambers	Right chambers
Intracavitary pediculated	Intramural/pericardial
Size <5 cm	Size >5 cm
Well defined limits	Infiltration/displacement of structures
Homogenous aspect	Heterogeneous aspect
Not perfused	Irregularly perfused
Without delayed contrast enhancement	Delayed irregular contrast enhancement
No other associated findings	Pericardial/Pleural effusion

the mass is also helpful (see Table 5.3). Although cardiac masses of different origin may share the same CMR features, meaning that the technique does not always allow their distinction, the predominant features of one or another type are worth studying as they may give more weight to a particular identification (see Table 5.4).

5.3 Benign Tumours and Masses

A mass with regular, non-infiltrative borders and high signal intensity in a *T1w-TSE* sequence is characteristically a lipoma (see Fig. 5.1, arrow). It is useful to compare its signal intensity with that of the subcutaneous fat, which should be similar. The signal is low in *T2w-TSE* sequences and is suppressed in *STIR* with fat saturation. There is no increase in signal after the administration of contrast, and it shows no delayed enhancement in *IR* sequences.

On the other hand, a signal of very low intensity in *T1w-TSE*, but which is very bright (high intensity) in T2, is characteristic of serous fluid; if a mass with these features is found in contact with the pericardium, particularly at the cardiophrenic angle, the diagnosis will, in all probability, be of a pericardial cyst (see Chap. 4, Fig. 4.7).

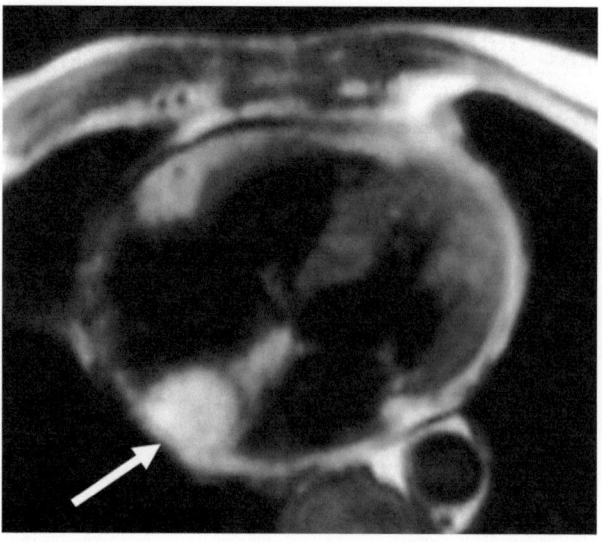

Fig. 5.1 T1w-TSE sequence on a transverse plane in a case of interatrial septal lipoma showing its characteristic bright signal (*arrow*)

A mass with intermediate level intensities in *T1w-TSE* may correspond to different processes, such as a myxoma (see Fig. 5.2, upper left panel), the most common primary tumour. A myxoma usually presents as a pedunculated, intracavitary atrial mass, although the extent of the base of implantation may vary. Its signal intensity is not necessarily homogenous, as it may present with areas of haemorrhage or calcification, but, in general, signal intensity is high in *T2w-TSE* (see Fig. 5.2, upper right panel) and also in *T1w-TSE* after contrast, which proves the vascularisation of the mass (see Fig. 5.2, lower left panel). There is usually delayed enhancement in *IR-TFE* sequences, not infrequently of heterogeneous distribution, indicating the presence of areas of necrosis or calcification (see Fig. 5.2, lower right panel).

The study of an intracavitary mass usually leads to differential diagnosis with thrombus, the most common mass in this location. For this, we first have to consider the presence of coexistent cardiac abnormalities, such as ventricular aneurysm or chamber dilatation due to valvular heart disease, which may promote the formation of thrombus. Also important are the morphological and dynamic features of the mass in cine-MR sequences: a chronic thrombus usually has a sessile base of implantation and regular borders (Fig. 5.3, arrows); a thrombus of recent origin may have more irregular borders and a more or less wide base of implantation, which may also be pedunculated and mobile (Fig. 5.4, arrow). A thrombus shows low signal intensity in *T1w-T1* and *T2* sequences, and for its identification, it is useful to observe the time course of contrast on a first-pass perfusion exam: an increase in the signal intensity of a mass during the first pass of contrast means that it is vascularised and perfused, while if there is no signal, the interpretation favours an avascular mass, such as a thrombus (Fig. 5.5, arrow). Finally, in *IR-TFE* sequences for the study of delayed enhancement, a thrombus will not enhance (see Fig. 5.6, black arrow), in contrast to scarred myocardium in the case of a post-infarction aneurysm with an intracavitary thrombus (see Fig. 5.6, white arrows).

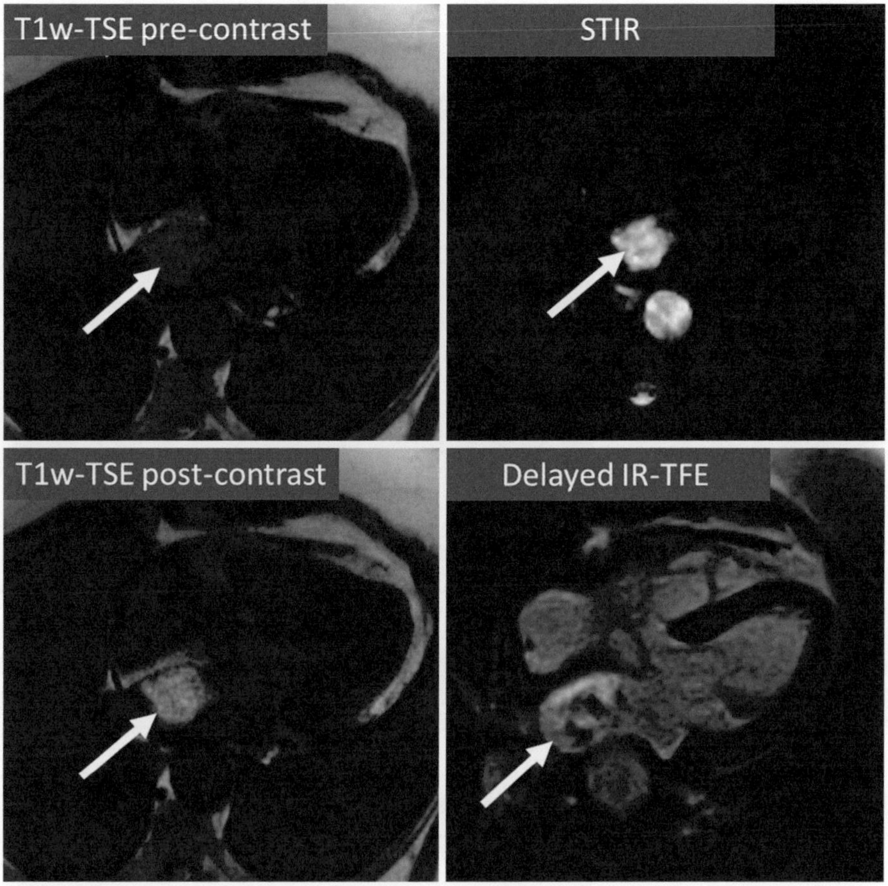

Fig. 5.2 Four-chamber planes with different sequences in a case of left atrial myxoma (*arrows*) (see text for explanation)

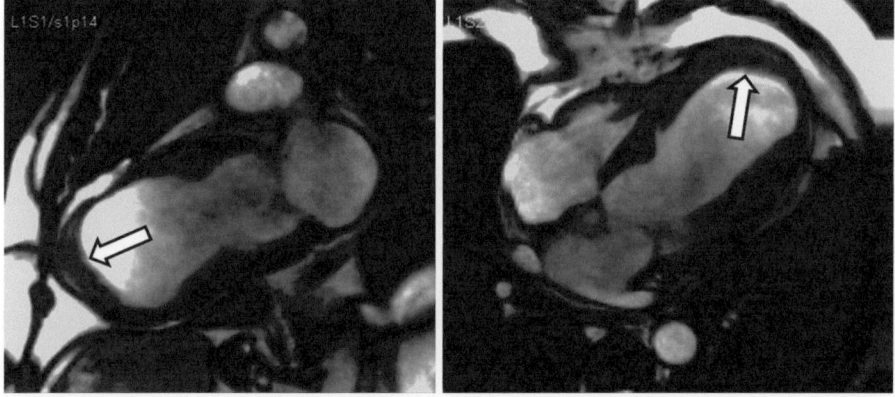

Fig. 5.3 Longitudinal planes from SSFP cine sequences in a case of a mural thrombus located at the left ventricular apical region (*arrows*)

Fig. 5.4 SSFP cine sequence on four-chamber plane showing a pedunculated, free-mobile thrombus in the right ventricle (*arrow*)

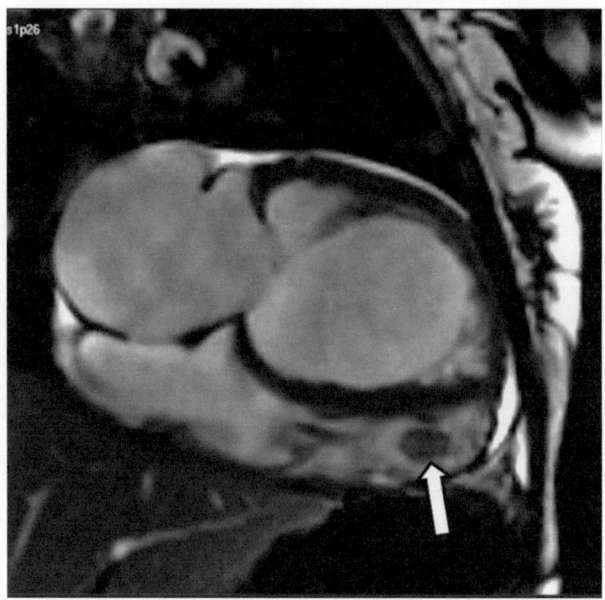

Fig. 5.5 Frame from a first-pass perfusion sequence showing lack of contrast enhancement of a mural left ventricular thrombus (*arrow*)

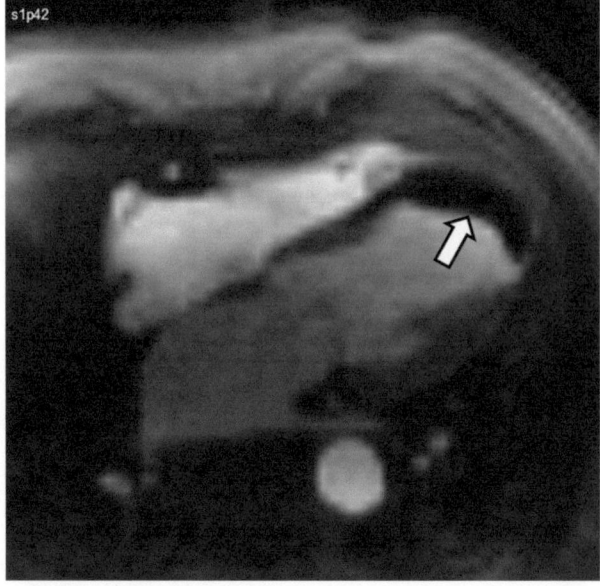

Fig. 5.6 IR-TFE sequence on four-chamber plane in a case of antero-apical infarction (*white arrows*) showing lack of delayed contrast enhancement of a large thrombotic mass lodged at the apical region (*black arrow*)

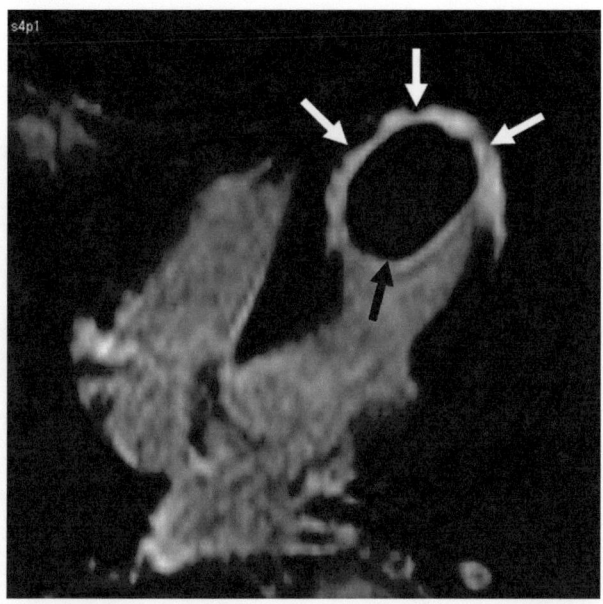

5.4 Primary Malignant Tumours

These are uncommon tumours, and among them the group of sarcomas stands out as the most often found. The characteristics of the tumour signal in the different sequences may not be distinct from those of benign tumours. A mass of sarcomatous origin may present with intermediate signal intensity in T1 (see Fig. 5.7, upper left panel), increased in T2 (see Fig. 5.7, upper right panel) and irregular contrast perfusion (see Fig. 5.7, lower left panel), as well as heterogeneous delayed enhancement (see Fig. 5.7, lower right panel). It is for this reason that other data must be assessed, such as rapid growth, which produces heterogeneous signal as it includes areas of necrosis or haemorrhage, irregular borders and infiltration of neighbouring structures, such as the pericardium, which leads to an accompanying effusion.

5.5 Pericardial Tumours

Among pericardial tumours, secondary metastasis of breast and lung cancer, melanoma, leukaemia or lymphoma is much more common than primary tumours, such as mesothelioma, which presents with irregular pericardial

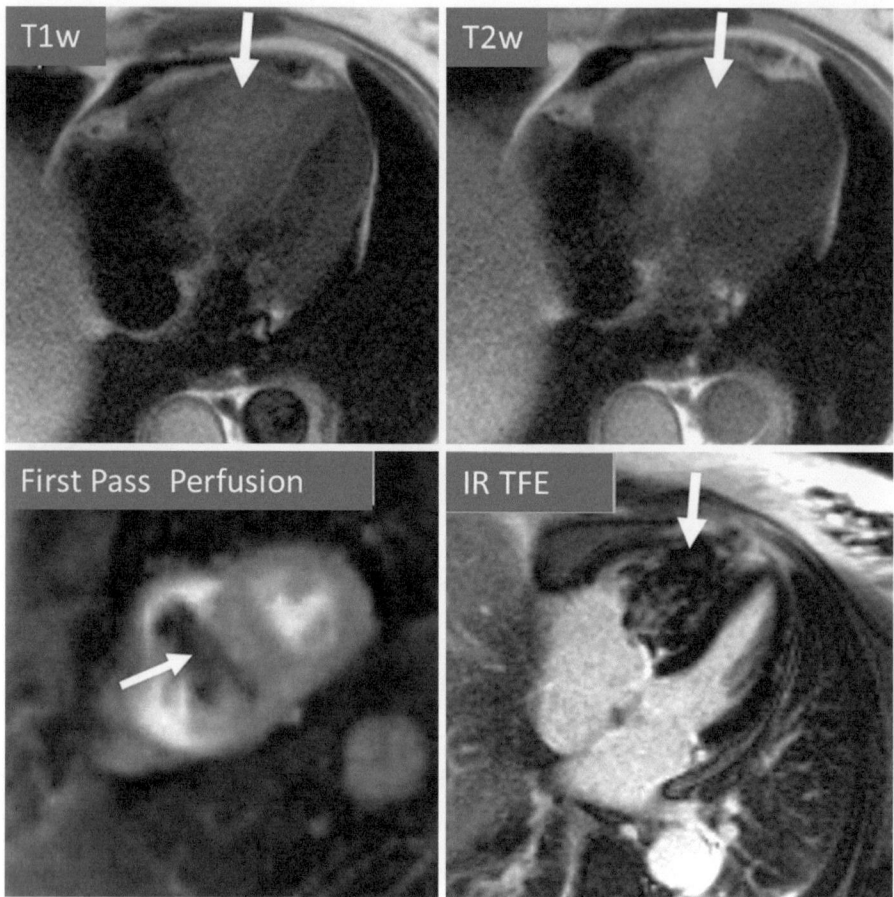

Fig. 5.7 Planes with different sequences in a case of left ventricular sarcoma (*arrows*) (see text for explanation)

thickening with heterogeneous signal (see Fig. 5.8, arrows), frequently with pleural involvement. The pericardial effusion that commonly accompanies malign pericardial tumours is frequently haematic in content. In this sense, it is important to know that the characteristics of the collection signal or of the haematic effusion vary with time, depending on the degree of degradation of the haemoglobin. In Table 5.5, the signal characteristics of blood collection are shown when analysed with T1 and T2 sequences, depending on the time elapsed. This analysis is useful when we wish to distinguish between acute and chronic haemorrhagic content.

Fig. 5.8 T1w-TSE sequence on a transverse plane showing areas of irregular pericardial increased thickness and infiltration with heterogeneous signal intensity (*arrows*) in a patient with malignant, secondary pericardial tumour

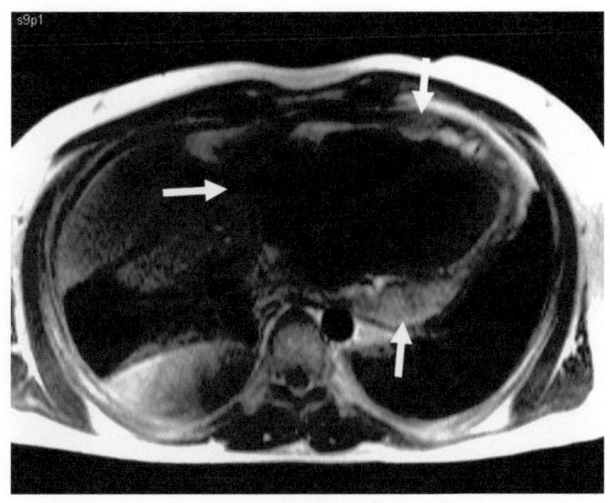

Table 5.5 Characterisation of haematic content by CMR

Stage	Date	Haemoglobin status	T1w	T2w
Acute	<24 h	Oxyhaemoglobin	Intermediate	Intermediate
Early subacute	3–4 days	Deoxyhaemoglobin	High	Intermediate
Late subacute	4–14 days	Methaemoglobin	Intermediate	High
Chronic	>14 days	Haemosiderin	Low	Low

5.6 Secondary Malignant Cardiac Tumours

Cardiac metastatic tumours occur much more frequently than primary ones, and among them pericardial infiltration by direct extension of pulmonary, mediastinal or lymphoma tumours stands out, along with infiltration of the left ventricle by invasion from the pulmonary veins (see Fig. 5.9, arrow) and the implantation of metastasis (see Fig. 5.10, white arrow).

5.7 Diagnosis of Non-tumoural Masses or Pseudomasses

Thanks to its wide field of view and excellent tissue contrast, MR is especially useful for clarifying the diagnosis of radiological images or echocardiograms that may be confused with tumoural processes, which are in fact due to non-tumour structures, the most frequent being hiatal hernia, epicardial fat and

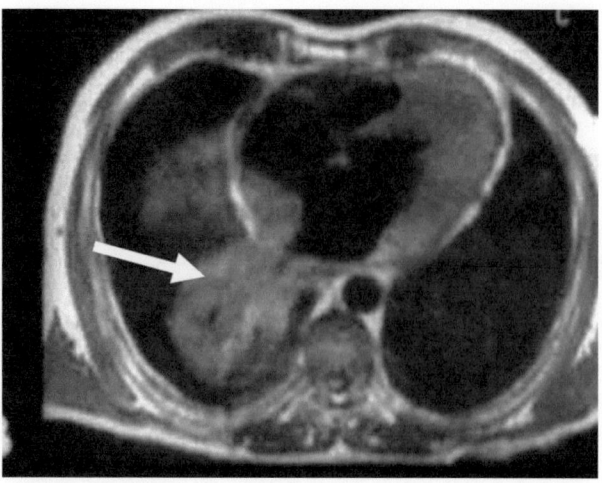

Fig. 5.9 T1w-TSE sequence in a patient with malignant lung carcinoma extended to the heart through the pulmonary veins (*arrow*)

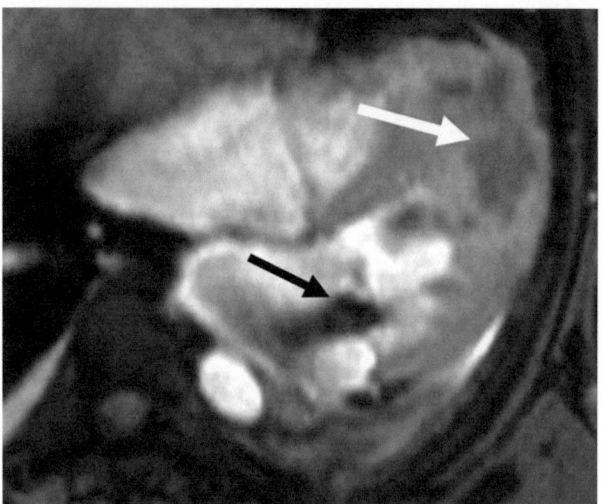

Fig. 5.10 Frame from an SSFP cine sequence on four-chamber plane showing metastatic myocardial masses (*white arrow*). A signal void is also seen due to significant mitral regurgitation (*black arrow*), probably secondary to distortion of the left ventricular myocardium and papillary muscles by the neoplastic process

pericardial cysts. It also helps to establish the diagnosis of what are known as cardiac "pseudomasses", which are, to say, normal heart structures that produce a cardiac mass image, such as the *crista terminalis* in the right atrium (see Fig. 5.11, arrow).

Fig. 5.11 Frame from an SSFP cine sequence centred on the atria and showing a prominent *crista terminalis* adjacent to the right atrial wall (*arrow*)

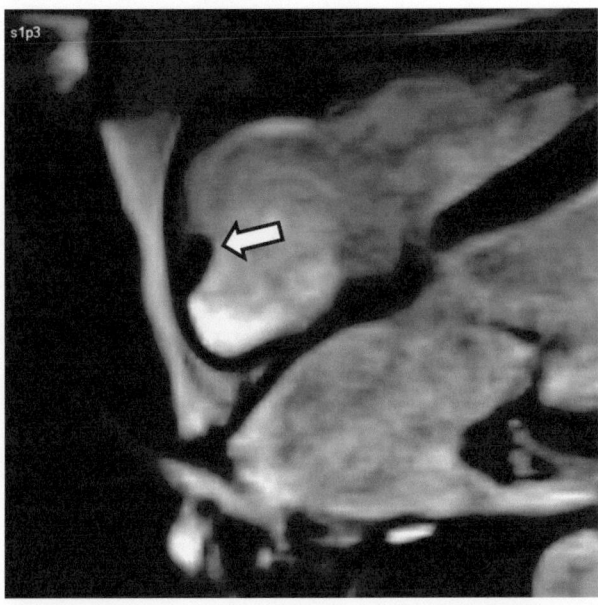

Recommended Bibliography

1. Fussen S, de Boeck BWL, Zellweger MJ, Bremerich J, Goetschalckx K, Zuber M et al (2011) Cardiovascular magnetic resonance imaging for diagnosis and clinical management of suspected cardiac masses and tumours. Eur Heart J 32:1551–1560
2. Hoey ETD, Shahid M, Ganeshan A, Baijal S, Simpson H, Watkin RW (2014) MRI assessment of cardiac tumors: part 1, multiparametric imaging protocols and spectrum of appearances of histologically benign lesions. Quant Imaging Med Surg 4:478–488
3. Hoey ETD, Shahid M, Ganeshan A, Baijal S, Simpson H, Watkin RW (2014) MRI assessment of cardiac tumors: part 2, spectrum of appearances of histologically malignant lesions and tumour mimics. Quant Imaging Med Surg 4:489–497
4. Motwani M, Kidambi A, Herzog BA, Uddin A, Greenwood JP, Plein S (2013) MR imaging of cardiac tumors and masses: a review of methods and clinical applications. Radiology 268:26–43
5. O'Donnell DH, Abbara S, Chaithiraphan V, Yared K, Killeen RP, Cury RC et al (2009) Cardiac tumors: optimal cardiac MR sequences and spectrum of imaging appearances. Am J Roentgenol 193:377–387

CMR Study Protocol for Great Vessels

6

Guillem Pons-Lladó

6.1 Introduction

Magnetic resonance is a highly appropriate technique for the study of the great vessels, in which its distinct modalities find application according to the specific disease.

Not all the processes that involve the great vessels fall within the domain of cardiac imaging, as some of them, such as the pulmonary thromboembolism, are, in general, not dealt with in the field of cardiology. For this reason, in this chapter, we will refer to those instances involving those structures in which cardiovascular magnetic resonance (CMR) is currently applied.

6.2 Study of the Thoracic Aorta

6.2.1 Aortic Aneurysm

The most common indication for a CMR study among acquired diseases of the thoracic aorta is the diagnosis of dilation or aneurysm, or its follow-up. Although a contrast MR angiography is an option, we believe that most of the cases with segmental aortic dilatation are adequately studied with *balanced-FFE* cine sequences guided by the following protocol:

1. Localising standard planes on axial, sagittal and coronal orientations, as usual.
2. A coronal cine sequence is prescribed aligned on axial localiser images encompassing the region of the left ventricular outflow tract, the aortic root and, if

---

G. Pons-Lladó, MD, PhD
Cardiac Imaging Unit, Cardiology Department, Hospital de la Santa Creu i Sant Pau,
Universitat Autònoma de Barcelona, Barcelona, Spain
e-mail: gpons@santpau.cat

© Springer International Publishing Switzerland 2016
G. Pons-Lladó (ed.), *Protocols for Cardiac MR and CT*,
DOI 10.1007/978-3-319-30831-9_6

possible, the ascending portion of the vessel (see Fig. 6.1, left panel). The resulting oblique coronal plane corresponds to a longitudinal section of the aortic root and the ascending portion (see Fig. 6.1, right panel).
3. A sagittal cine sequence is aligned over the cine image obtained at the previous step (see Fig. 6.2, left panel). The resultant sagittal oblique plane is again a longitudinal slice that is orthogonal to the previous (see Fig. 6.2, right panel).
4. A cine sequence with double angulation over the two previous planes is localised transversal to the aortic root (see Fig. 6.3, left panel). We obtain, thus, a cross-sectional plane of the vessel at this level (see Fig. 6.3, right panel) in

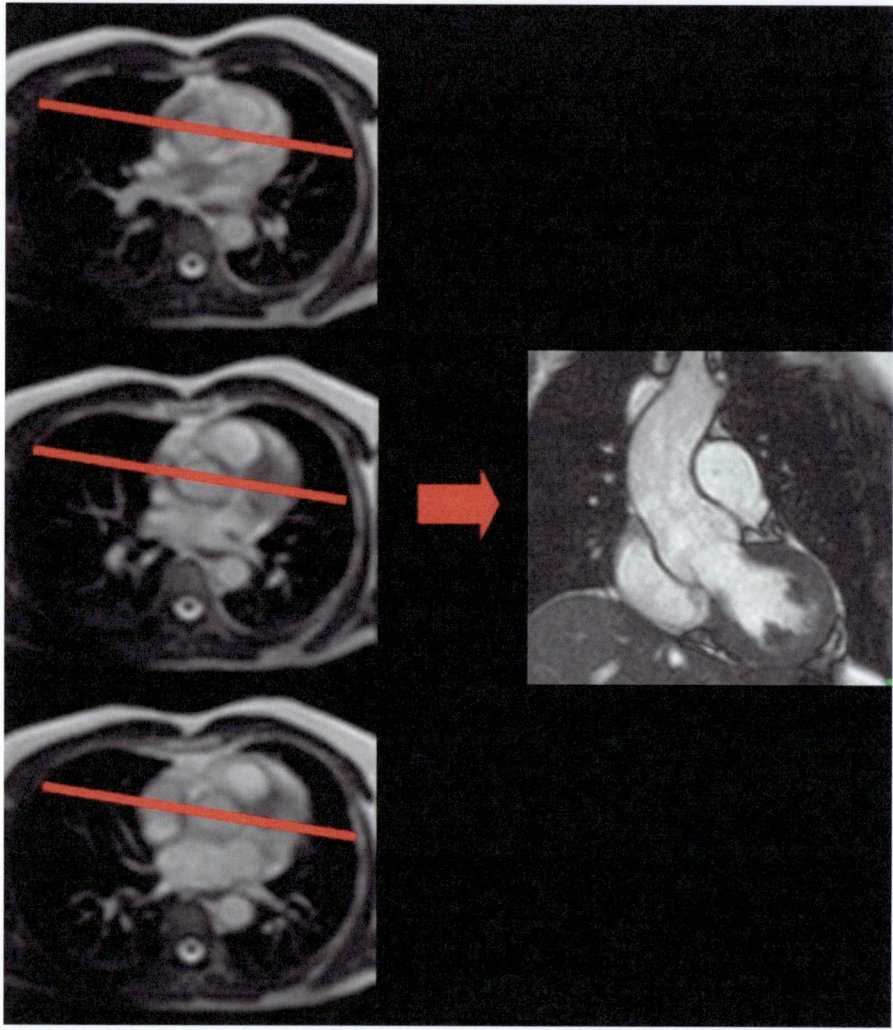

Fig. 6.1 Prescription of an SSFP cine sequence on axial localiser slices (*red lines, on panels of the left column*) and the resultant plane (*right panel*), aligned on a longitudinal axis of the aortic root

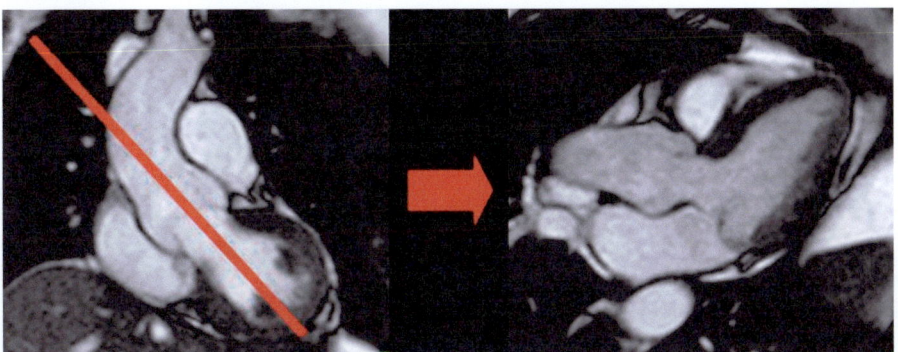

Fig. 6.2 Prescription of a longitudinal plane of the aortic root (*right panel*) with an orthogonal orientation to that from Fig. 6.1 (*red line, on the left panel*)

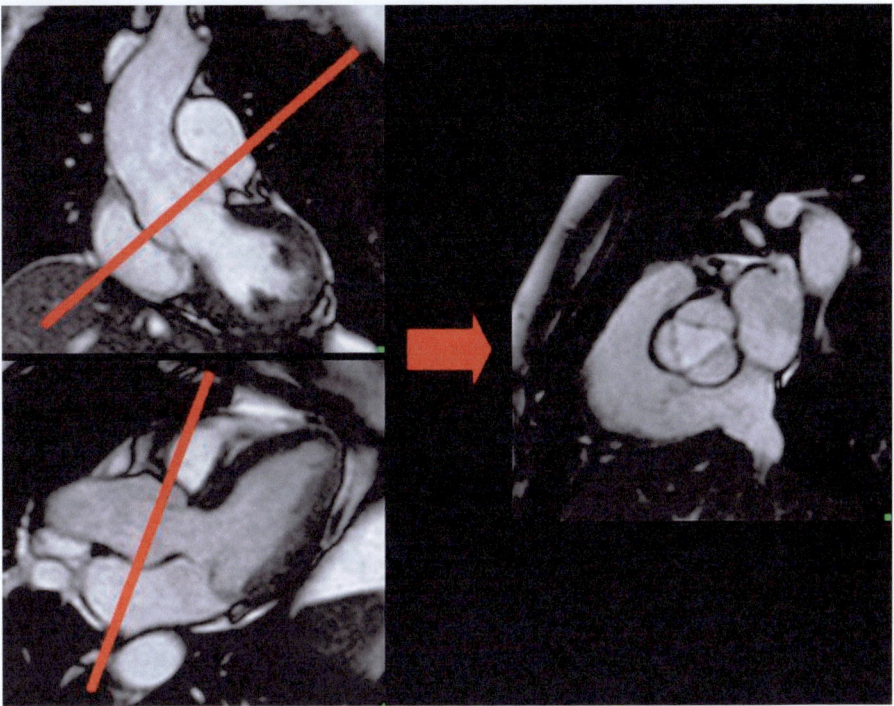

Fig. 6.3 SSFP cine sequence oriented on a cross-sectional plane of the aortic root (*right panel*) planned by double oblique angulation (*red lines*) on the longitudinal planes obtained in Figs. 6.1 and 6.2

which it is possible to determine the symmetry of the sinuses of Valsalva and to measure the maximal diameter of the aortic root, as well as studying, in the cine sequence, the morphology of the aortic valve and its function. Any abnormal dilatation of the aortic root, whether global or localised, is detected (see Fig. 6.4,

Fig. 6.4 SSFP cine sequence oriented on a cross-sectional plane of the aortic root where a bicuspid aortic valve is seen (*black arrow*) and, also, an aneurysm of the left coronary sinus of Valsalva (*white arrow*)

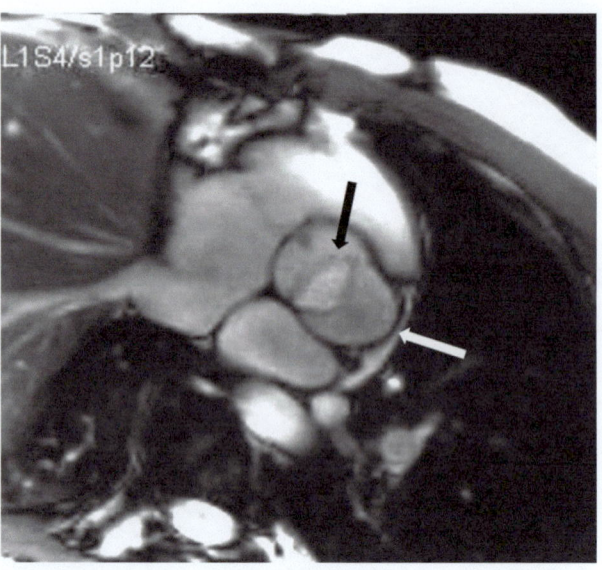

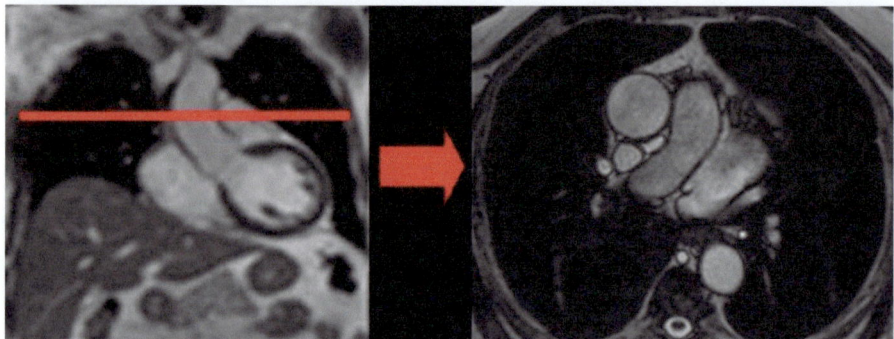

Fig. 6.5 Prescription of an SSFP cine sequence on a coronal localiser slice (*red line on the left panel*) and the resultant plane (*right panel*), aligned on cross-sectional views of the ascending and descending aorta

white arrow), and a careful exam of the aortic leaflets is also easily performed, this being particularly useful for identifying a bicuspid aortic valve (see Fig. 6.4, black arrow).
5. The standardisation of the measurements in the study of the thoracic aorta requires an additional cine sequence to be performed, in this case with a strict transversal orientation at the level of the pulmonary artery trunk (see Fig. 6.5, left panel) to obtain a cross-sectional plane of the aorta in its ascending and descending segments (see Fig. 6.5, right panel), where these measurements must be performed.

6 CMR Study Protocol for Great Vessels

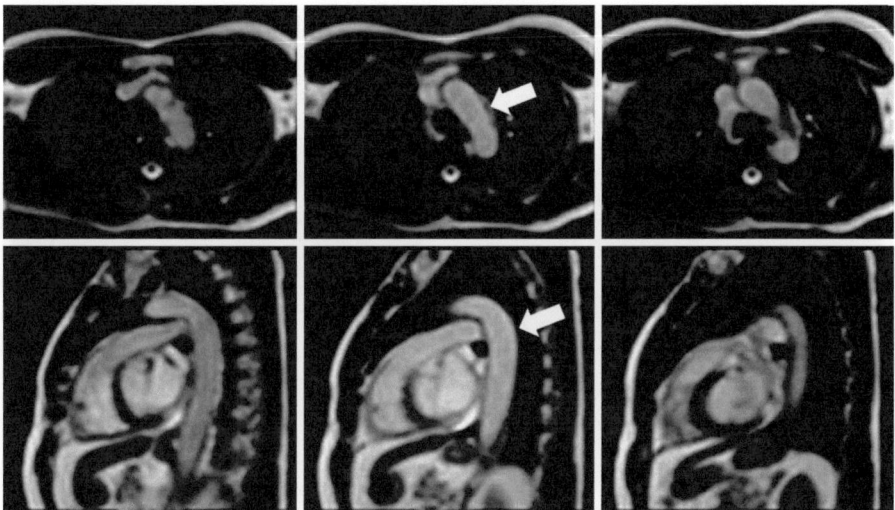

Fig. 6.6 Series of transverse (*upper row*) and sagittal (*lower row*) localiser planes where the region of the arch and the descending thoracic aorta may be seen (*arrows*)

6. The examination of the aortic arch and the proximal descending aorta is made on the axial and sagittal localiser planes themselves (see arrows in Fig. 6.6), and, in case of abnormal findings, then additional oriented cine sequences may be added.

This study protocol provides with images on which reliable measures may be obtained at every segment of the thoracic aorta (i.e. aortic root, sino-tubular junction, ascending, arch and descending portions) and constitutes thus an appropriate reference for future follow-up studies, in cases of acquired aortic aneurysm. However, in those cases where there is irregular or distorted enlargement of the vessel, a conventional MR contrast angiography with potential for 3D reconstruction must be performed (see Fig. 6.7).

6.2.2 Aortic Dissection

Aortic dissection requires always an MR angiogram study which allows the true lumen of the vessel to be identified by the high intensity of its signal (see Fig. 6.8, white arrow), as well as the false one, with lower signal intensity (see Fig. 6.8, black arrow) and its characteristics, such as the presence of thrombosis, which causes absence of contrast in the false lumen (see Fig. 6.8, asterisk).

The individual slices of the whole angiographic study must be carefully examined as this may allow the detection of an intimal tear of the aortic wall (see arrows in Fig. 6.9). As CMR is frequently used in the follow-up of patients with repaired dissection, and the main concern in these cases is progressive aortic dilatation, a precise measurement of the vessel diameter at the standard levels mentioned above is particularly important.

Fig. 6.7 3D reconstruction of a contrast MR angiography of the aorta in a case of aneurysm of the ascending aorta (*arrow*)

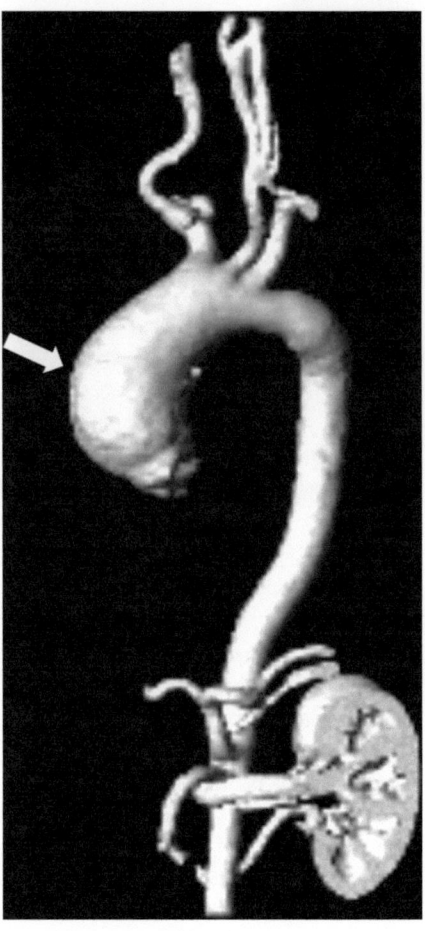

The clinical suspicion of aortic wall pathology without intimal tear, such as intramural haematoma, requires a morphological study with T1w-TSE sequences in multiple slices on axial planes, in which an abnormal wall thickening may be detected (see Fig. 6.10, arrow).

6.3 Study of Pulmonary Veins

The increasing use of ablation procedures on the pulmonary veins has stimulated interest in imaging methods for the evaluation of these vessels. The MR contrast angiography of the pulmonary veins is performed with coronal orientation of the planes of the sequence (see Fig. 6.11, left panel). The resulting images can be analysed on the angiographic slices themselves (see Fig. 6.11, central panel) or in 3D reconstructions (see Fig. 6.11, right panel).

Fig. 6.8 MIP reconstruction of a contrast MR angiography of the aorta in a case of dissection showing the true lumen (*white arrow*) and the false one (*black arrow*), with an area of dark signal intensity (*asterisk*) suggesting thrombosis of the false lumen

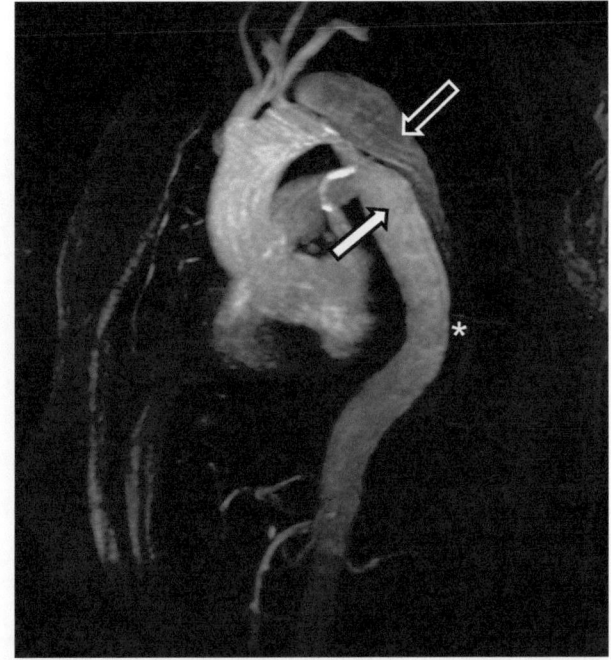

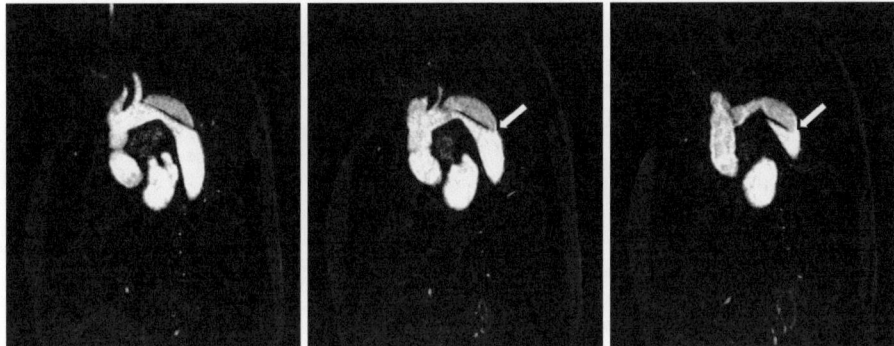

Fig. 6.9 Slices from a contrast MR angiography in a case of dissection showing an intimal tear of the aortic wall (*arrows*)

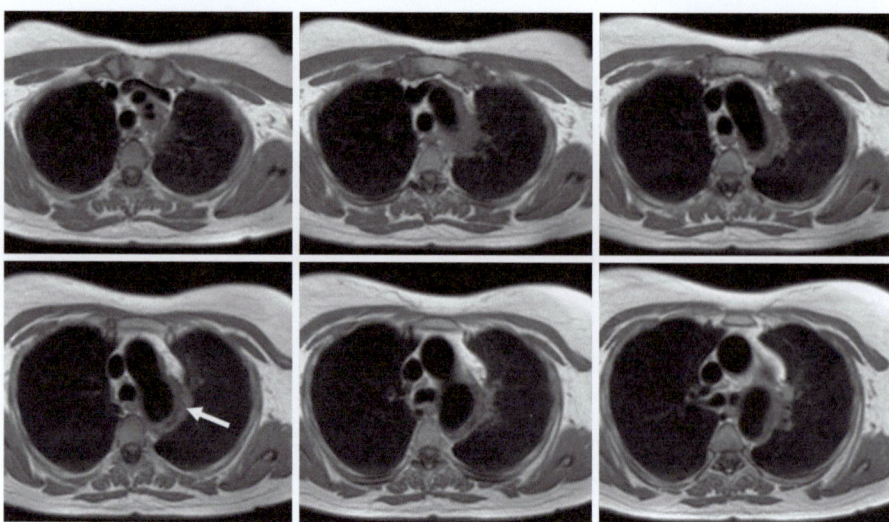

Fig. 6.10 T1w-TSE sequence on transverse planes showing increased aortic wall thickness with a homogeneous, intermediate signal intensity due to intramural hematoma

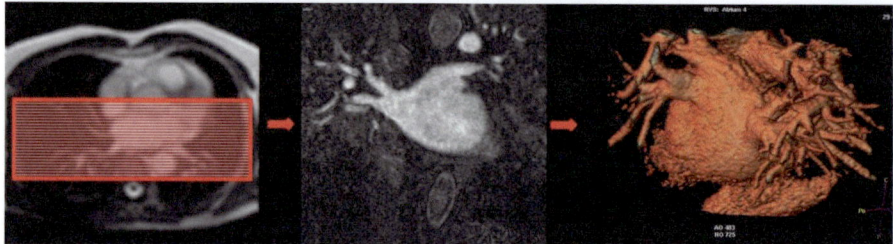

Fig. 6.11 MR contrast angiography of the pulmonary veins: planning of the stack of slices on a transverse localiser plane (*red lines on the left panel*), one of the resultant slices (*centre panel*) and 3D reconstruction of the whole study (*right panel*)

Recommended Bibliography

1. Davies AE, Lewandowski AJ, Holloway CJ, Ntusi NAB, Banerjee R, Nethononda R et al (2014) Observational study of regional aortic size referenced to body size: production of a cardiovascular magnetic resonance nomogram. J Cardiovasc Magn Reson 16:9
2. Grotenhuis HB, de Roos A (2011) Structure and function of the aorta in inherited and congenital heart disease and the role of MRI. Heart 97:66–74
3. Litmanovich D, Bankier AA, Cantin L, Raptopoulos V, Boiselle PM (2009) CT and MRI in diseases of the aorta. Am J Roentgenol 193:928–940

CMR Study Protocol for Valvular Diseases

Francesc Carreras and Guillem Pons-Lladó

7.1 Introduction

Doppler echocardiography is the technique of choice for the study of any type of valvular heart disease. Cardiovascular magnetic resonance (CMR), however, has resources for providing significant quantitative information that can be considered complementary to ultrasound.

All CMR strategies for the study of valvular diseases are based on *balanced TFE* cine sequences and on those of velocity mapping, or *phase contrast*. From each one, or from their combination, we can derive information on valvular morphology and dynamics, on ventricular volumes and function and on the regurgitant volume and regurgitant fraction (RF) in the case of valvular insufficiencies.

7.2 Study of Atrio–ventricular Valve Regurgitations

7.2.1 Mitral Insufficiency

1. Once the usual localiser planes have been acquired, the study protocol begins with the complete longitudinal and short-axis *balanced TFE* cine series for the calculation of left ventricular volume and function (see Chap. 1, Figs. 1.3–1.7).
2. It is important to analyse the longitudinal cine sequences in motion in search for a signal of turbulent flow, which appears as an area of loss of signal intensity (signal void), which contrasts with the uniformly high signal intensity of the normal laminar flow (see Fig. 7.1, arrows). From the characteristics of the width, depth and extension of the signal void, some estimation of the degree of mitral

---

F. Carreras, MD, PhD • G. Pons-Lladó, MD, PhD (✉)
Cardiac Imaging Unit, Cardiology Department, Hospital de la Santa Creu i Sant Pau,
Universitat Autònoma de Barcelona, Barcelona, Spain
e-mail: gpons@santpau.cat

regurgitation can be made, although this cannot be considered as a reliable method for grading the lesion. In addition to the standard longitudinal cine sequences, it is recommended to acquire also slices with intermediate orientation in relation to the two- and four-chamber views (i.e. three-chamber plane) in order to reveal localised morphological abnormalities of the mitral valve, such as a prolapse of one of the leaflets (see Fig. 7.2, white arrow).

3. Next, a *phase contrast* sequence is acquired oriented on the plane of the ascending aorta (see Chap. 1, Fig. 1.24). From the area of the vessel traced over the images of magnitude, which the equipment transfers to the phase images (see Fig. 7.3, upper panels), the flow curve is obtained (see Fig. 7.3, lower panel) from which it is

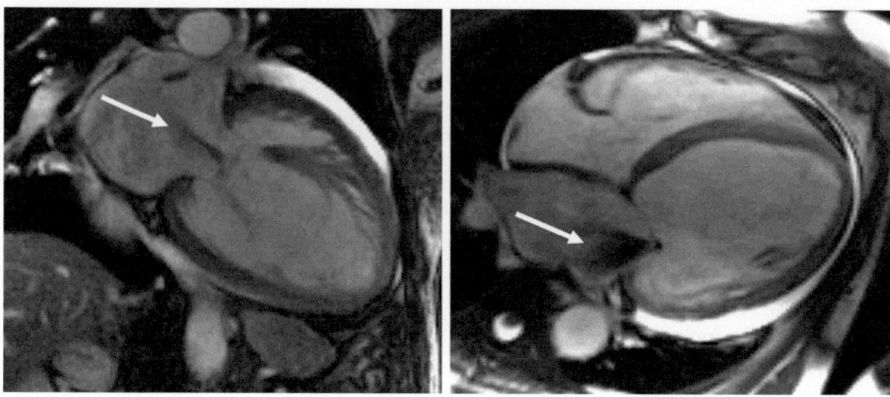

Fig. 7.1 Systolic frames from SSFP cine sequences on longitudinal planes in a patient with mitral regurgitation: a signal void is seen (*arrows*) indicating the area of the turbulent flow

Fig. 7.2 Systolic frame from an SSFP cine sequence on a longitudinal three-chamber plane in a patient with mitral valve prolapse of the posterior leaflet (*white arrow*) and secondary mitral regurgitation with an eccentric jet (*black arrow*)

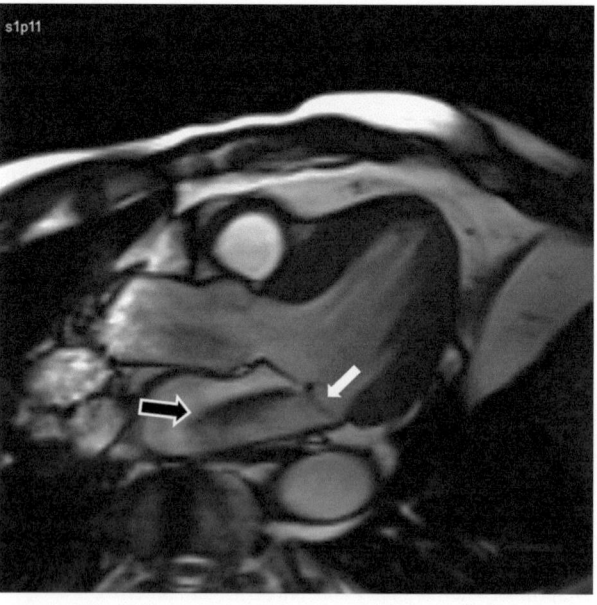

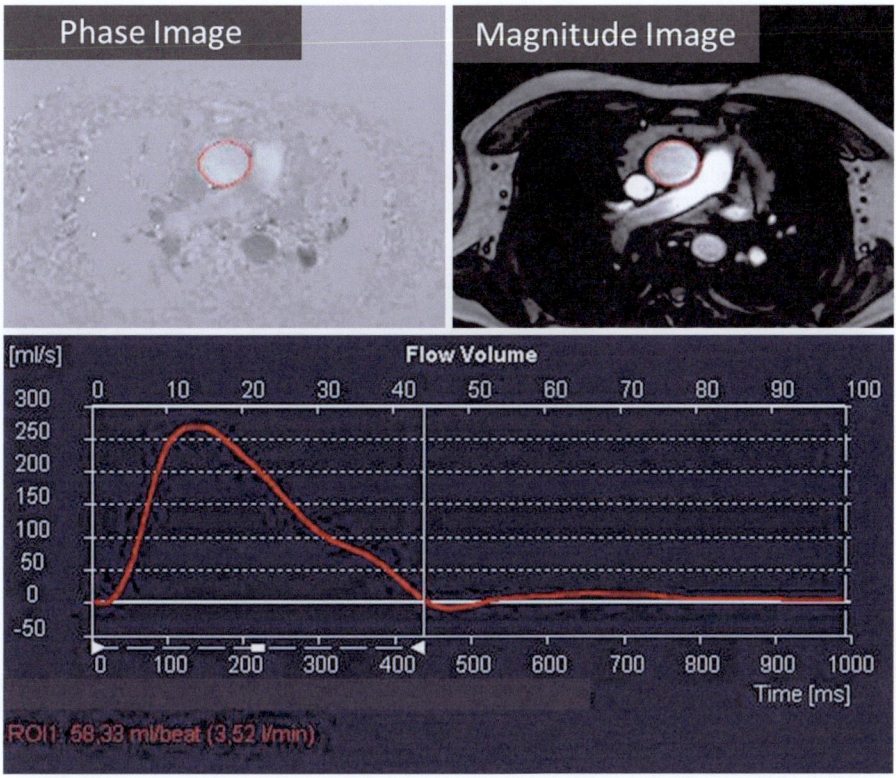

Fig. 7.3 Phase contrast sequence oriented on a transverse plane of the ascending aorta (*upper panels*) and the resultant flow curve (*lower panel*), where the systolic volume has been estimated

possible to calculate the aortic systolic volume. The estimate of the mitral regurgitant volume is derived by subtracting the aortic systolic volume from the total left ventricular stroke volume, which is calculated on the series of multiple planes on the ventricular short axis (see Chap. 1, Fig. 1.10). In case of valve insufficiency, the mitral RF is estimated as the regurgitant volume divided by the left ventricular stroke volume. Mild regurgitation is considered to be present when the RF <15%, mild to moderate if the RF is 16–25%, moderately severe if it is 26–45% and definitively important when RF >45%. For this calculation to be reliable, it is necessary to accurately measure the left ventricular volume at both end-diastole and end-systole, taking special care in the tracing of endocardial borders, particularly at the most basal slices of the short-axis cine sequences (see Chap. 1, Fig. 1.11).

7.2.2 Tricuspid Insufficiency

The presence of tricuspid insufficiency also creates a flow turbulence which causes a signal void in *balanced TFE* sequences on a four-chamber longitudinal plane (see Fig. 7.4, arrow). It is necessary, for its quantification, to perform the

Fig. 7.4 Systolic frame from an SSFP cine sequence on four-chamber plane in a patient with tricuspid regurgitation: a signal void is seen (*arrow*) indicating the turbulent flow

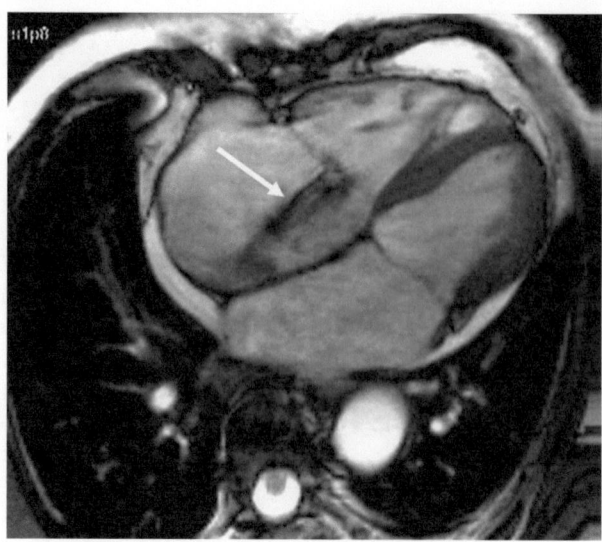

complete cine series on the ventricular short-axis planes, for the calculation, in this case, of the volumes of the right ventricle (see Chap. 1, Fig. 1.10), from which the right ventricular stroke volume is derived. In this case, the *phase contrast* sequences will be oriented orthogonally to the main pulmonary artery (see Chap. 1, Fig. 1.25), a cross-sectional plane of the vessel being thus obtained (see Fig. 7.5, upper panels) from which the pulmonary flow curve is derived (see Fig. 7.5, lower panel), and the systolic pulmonary volume is estimated. Thus, the tricuspid regurgitant volume is obtained by subtracting the systolic pulmonary volume from the right ventricular stroke volume and the tricuspid RF then calculated as the quotient between the regurgitant volume and the stroke volume.

7.3 Study of Sigmoid Valve Regurgitations

7.3.1 Aortic Insufficiency

1. The study protocol also begins with the complete longitudinal and short-axis *balanced TFE* cine series to obtain the calculations of left ventricular volume and function (see Chap. 1, Figs. 1.3–1.7).
2. An appropriate study of aortic valve regurgitation by CMR must include an examination of the thoracic aorta following the protocol described in Chap. 5, especially including the planes of the aortic valve, root and ascending portion (see Chap. 6, Figs. 6.1–6.3). The slices of the valve plane will allow the study of valve morphology and detection of a possible bicuspid aortic valve (see Fig. 7.6), while in the longitudinal slices oriented on the aortic valve plane, a signal void effect due to the turbulence of the aortic regurgitant flow (see Fig. 7.7, arrow)

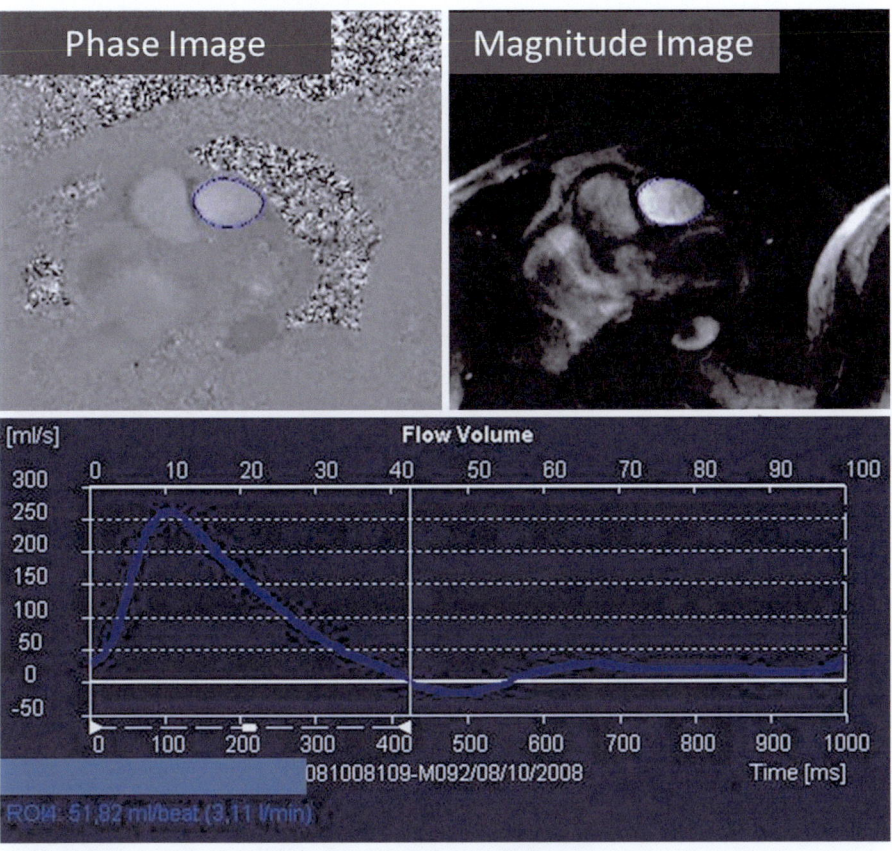

Fig. 7.5 Phase contrast sequence oriented on a transverse plane of the main pulmonary artery (*upper panels*) and the resultant flow curve (*lower panel*), where the systolic volume has been estimated

may appear, which is useful, as already mentioned, for the qualitative grading of the regurgitation.
3. Our study protocol of aortic regurgitation include *phase contrast* sequences at three levels:
   - First, at the sinotubular junction, the orientation of which is obtained by double angulation on the cine planes acquired previously of the root and the ascending aorta (see Fig. 7.8). This localization is where the velocity map is most sensitive for detecting the presence of a retrograde diastolic flow due to aortic valve insufficiency. The aortic regurgitant volume is determined here directly on the retrograde flow curve, and the RF is the relation between this and the antegrade systolic flow (see Fig. 7.9, lower panel). An aortic insufficiency is considered as mild when the RF is <10%, mild to moderate if it is 11–19%, moderately severe if it is from 20 to 29% and definitively significant when the RF is >30%.

Fig. 7.6 Systolic frame from an SSFP cine sequence oriented on a cross-sectional plane of the aortic root in a case of bicuspid aortic valve. A fibrous raphe is seen indicating a congenital fusion of the coronary cusps (*arrow*)

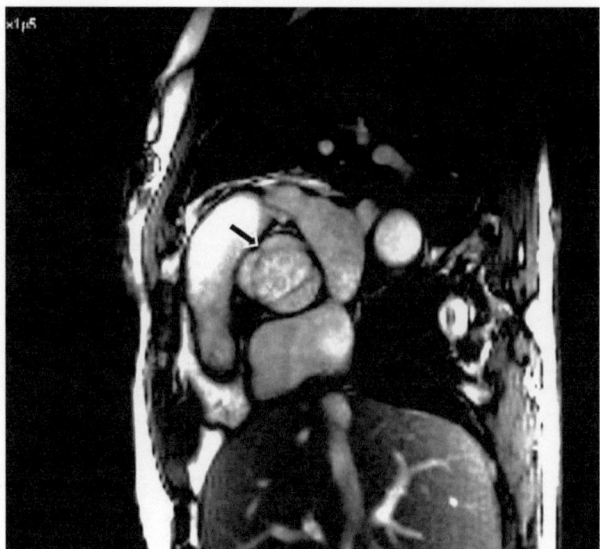

Fig. 7.7 Diastolic frame from an SSFP cine sequence on a longitudinal three-chamber plane in a patient with aortic regurgitation showing the signal void induced by the turbulent regurgitant flow (*arrow*)

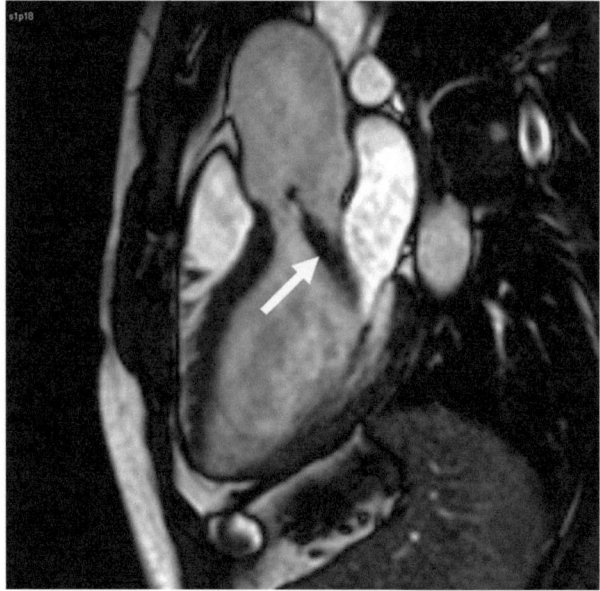

- Second, we perform a velocity map study at the level of the ascending aorta, on a strictly axial plane at the level of the main pulmonary artery (see Chap. 1, Fig. 1.24). On the ascending aorta, we trace the region of interest (see Fig. 7.10, black arrow on the upper panel) from which the aortic regurgitant volume is also detected (see Fig. 7.10, middle panel) and can be checked against that obtained at the sinotubular junction. This same plane also offers

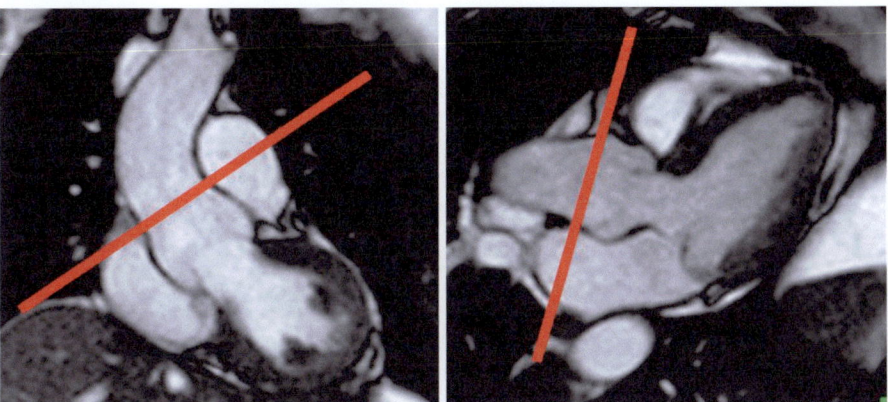

Fig. 7.8 Planning of a phase contrast study (*red lines*) at a cross-sectional level of the aortic sinotubular junction by double angulation on orthogonal longitudinal planes of the aortic root

the possibility to examine the descending thoracic aorta (see Fig. 7.10, white arrow on the upper panel), which velocity map (see Fig. 7.10, lower panel) contains information that is also relevant in the study of aortic insufficiency. Thus, the determination of a regurgitant volume at this level >10 ml of absolute value is indicative of aortic insufficiency of at least moderate in degree, while the observation of regurgitant holodiastolic flow in the descending aorta is a sensitive and specific sign of severe aortic valve insufficiency

- Finally, it is also recommendable to determine the velocity map in the main pulmonary artery (see Fig. 7.5), in order to obtain the pulmonary systolic volume which, when compared with the aortic, serves as a double check, as it should agree with the effective aortic systolic volume (antegrade volume minus regurgitant volume).

7.3.2 Pulmonary Valve Insufficiency

Sigmoid pulmonary regurgitation is of interest, from the diagnostic point of view, in patients with certain surgically corrected forms of congenital heart disease, in particular in cases of tetralogy of Fallot. As with all studies of valve function, the complete cine series is performed on the short-axis ventricular planes to calculate the volumes of the right ventricle (see Chap. 1, Fig. 1.10). The *phase contrast* sequences are oriented orthogonally to the main pulmonary artery (see Chap. 1, Fig. 1.25), and from the flow curve obtained (see Fig. 7.11, right panel), the pulmonary RF is estimated. The regurgitation is considered as mild if the RF is $<20\,\%$, moderate when it is between 20 and 40 % and significant if it is $>40\,\%$.

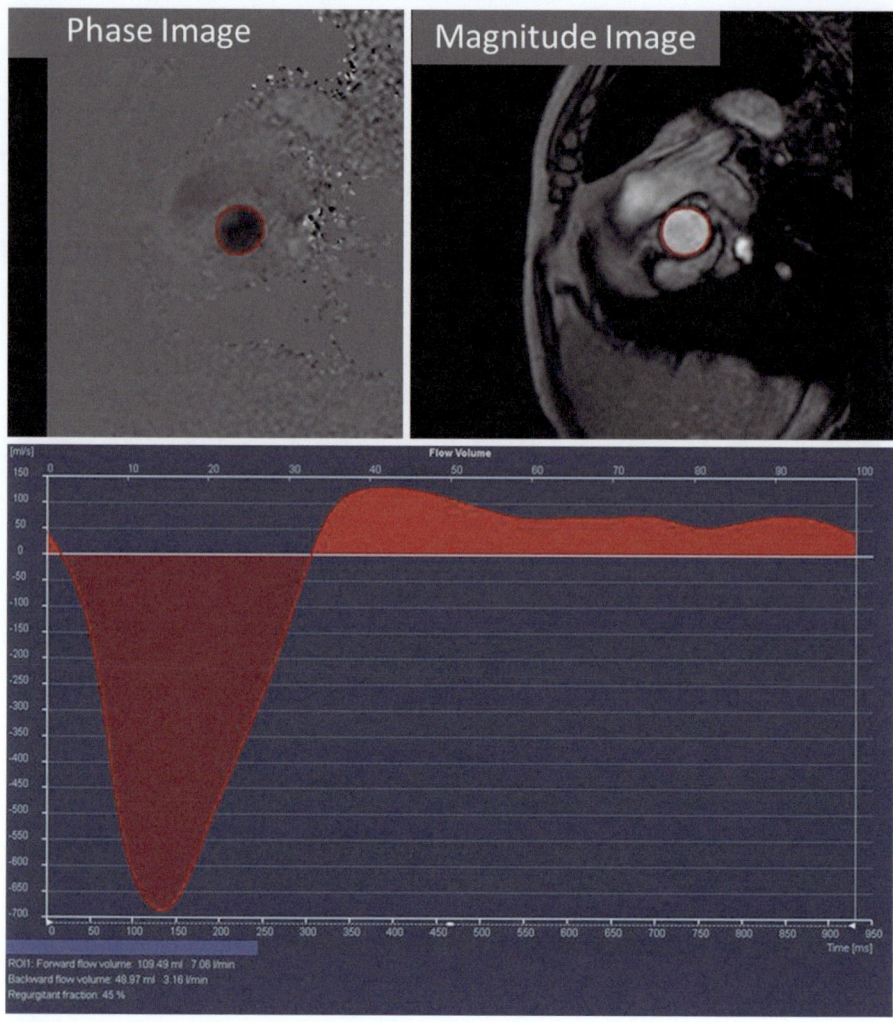

Fig. 7.9 Phase contrast study planned as in Fig. 7.8. The flow curve (*lower panel*) shows retrograde diastolic flow (*positive curve*) which corresponds to the aortic regurgitant volume

7.4 Study of Valvular Stenosis

Although CMR is at a disadvantage compared to Doppler echocardiography for the study of valvular stenosis, it is possible to obtain information both on the morphological and effective valvular area through *balanced TFE* cine sequences oriented on the valve plane (see arrow, on Fig. 7.12) and, also on flow velocity, by applying *phase contrast* sequences on a plane orthogonal to that of the direction of flow (through plane). The phase images of this sequence can reveal, on one side, the transvalvular flow contour, which reproduces the shape of the valve orifice, such as

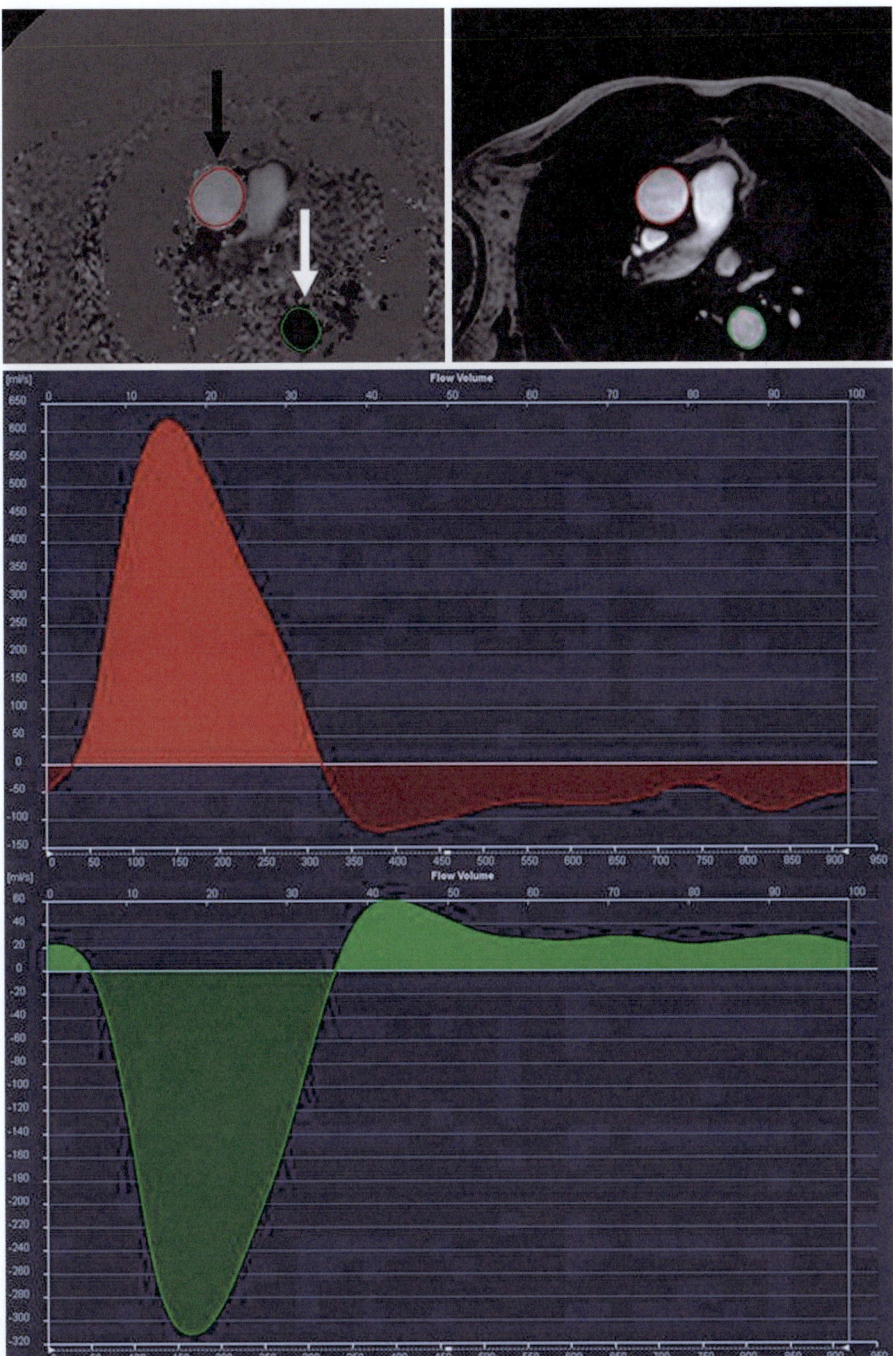

Fig. 7.10 Phase contrast study planned on a transverse plane containing cross-sectional views of both the ascending (*black arrow*) and descending (*white arrow*) segments of the thoracic aorta. A diastolic retrograde volume due to aortic regurgitation can be measured at both levels (*middle and lower panels*)

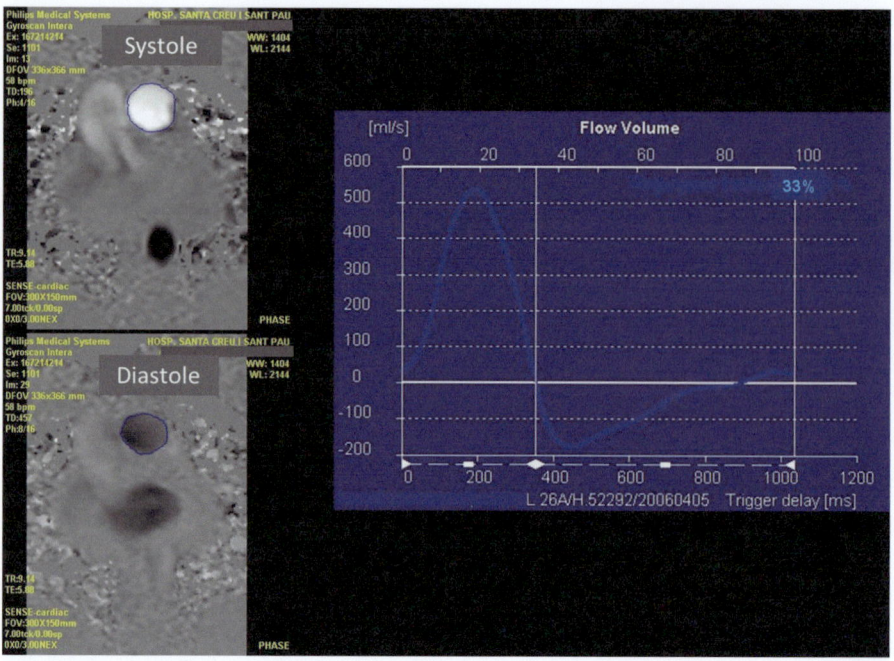

Fig. 7.11 Phase contrast study at the main pulmonary artery in a case of pulmonary insufficiency: systolic and diastolic frames of the sequence (*left panels*) show flow with opposite direction in each time interval (*bright vs. dark signal*, respectively). The resultant flow curve allows for the estimation of both antegrade and retrograde volume and, from its ratio, also the regurgitant fraction

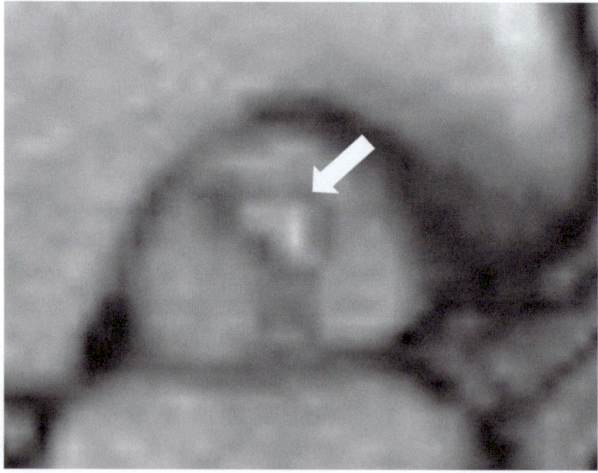

Fig. 7.12 Systolic frame from an SSFP cine sequence in a patient with aortic stenosis oriented on a cross-sectional plane of the valve where the maximal orifice area can be measured (*arrow*)

7 CMR Study Protocol for Valvular Diseases

in aortic stenosis due to a bicuspid valve (see Fig. 7.13, arrow on upper left panel), and, on the other side, may quantify the maximum transvalvular velocity (see Fig. 7.13, lower panel). If the velocity encoding (VENC) has been set at a value that is lower to that of the maximal blood velocity, an aliasing phenomenon is produced on the phase signal (see Fig. 7.14, arrow on the upper panel) which alters the flow curve (see Fig. 7.14a, arrow on lower panel). The VENC in this case must be increased until the aliasing signal disappears (see Fig. 7.14b).

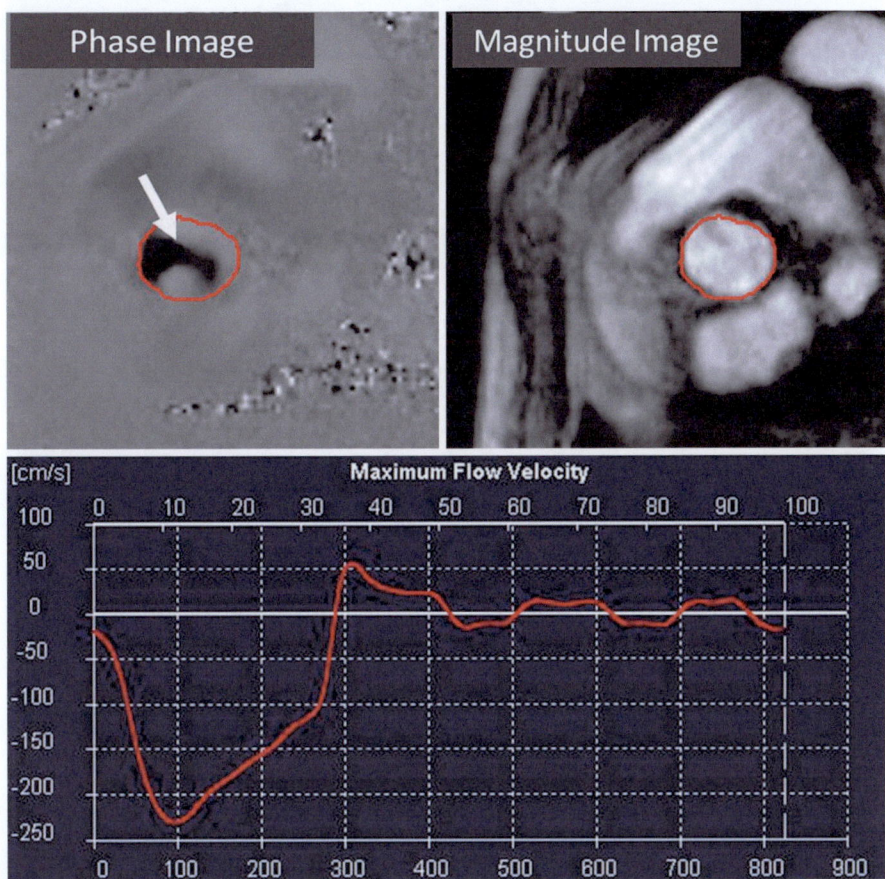

Fig. 7.13 Phase contrast study planned at the level of the sinotubular junction in a patient with aortic stenosis and bicuspid valve. The profile of the valve opening is seen at the phase images (*arrow*, in *left upper panel*), while the flow curve in a scale of blood velocity (*lower panel*) allows for the estimation of the maximal transvalvular gradient

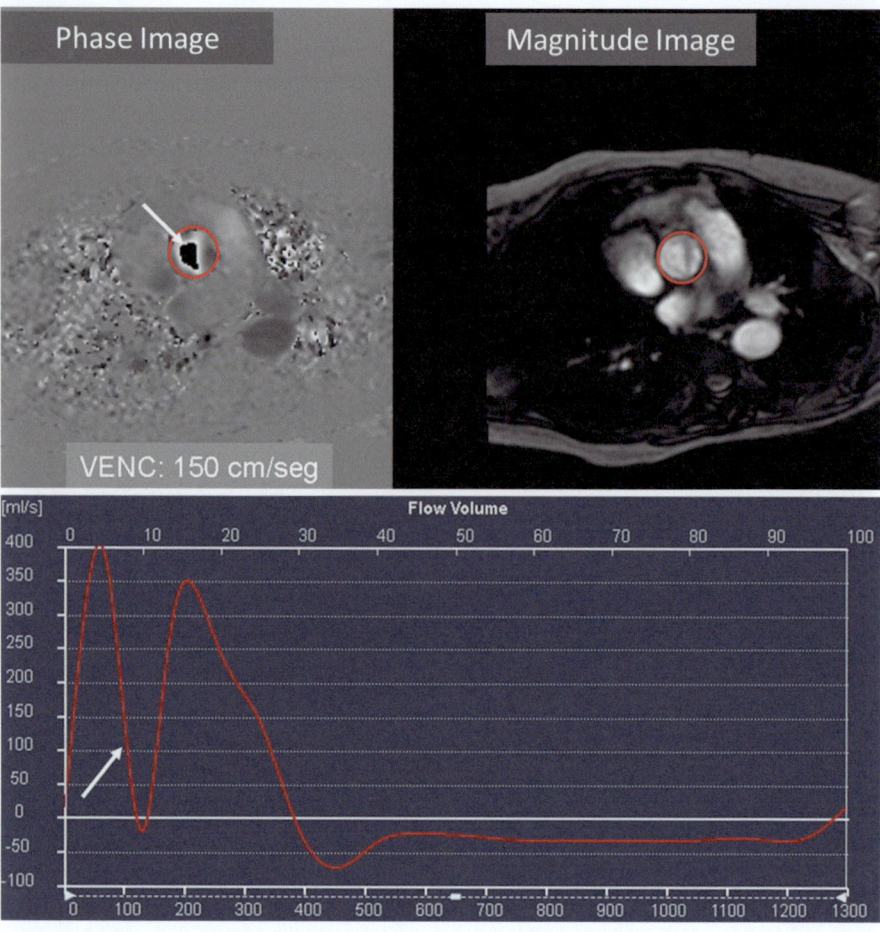

Fig. 7.14 (**a**) Phase contrast study at the level of the sinotubular junction in a patient with aortic stenosis showing an aliasing phenomenon (*arrow*, in the *left upper panel*) due to a VENC excessively low (150 cm/s), leading to a distorted flow curve (*arrow*, in *lower panel*). (**b**) The same study with an increased VENC (200 cm/s) shows disappearance of the aliasing effect and the artefact of the curve that allow for a reliable estimation of the flow volume

7 CMR Study Protocol for Valvular Diseases

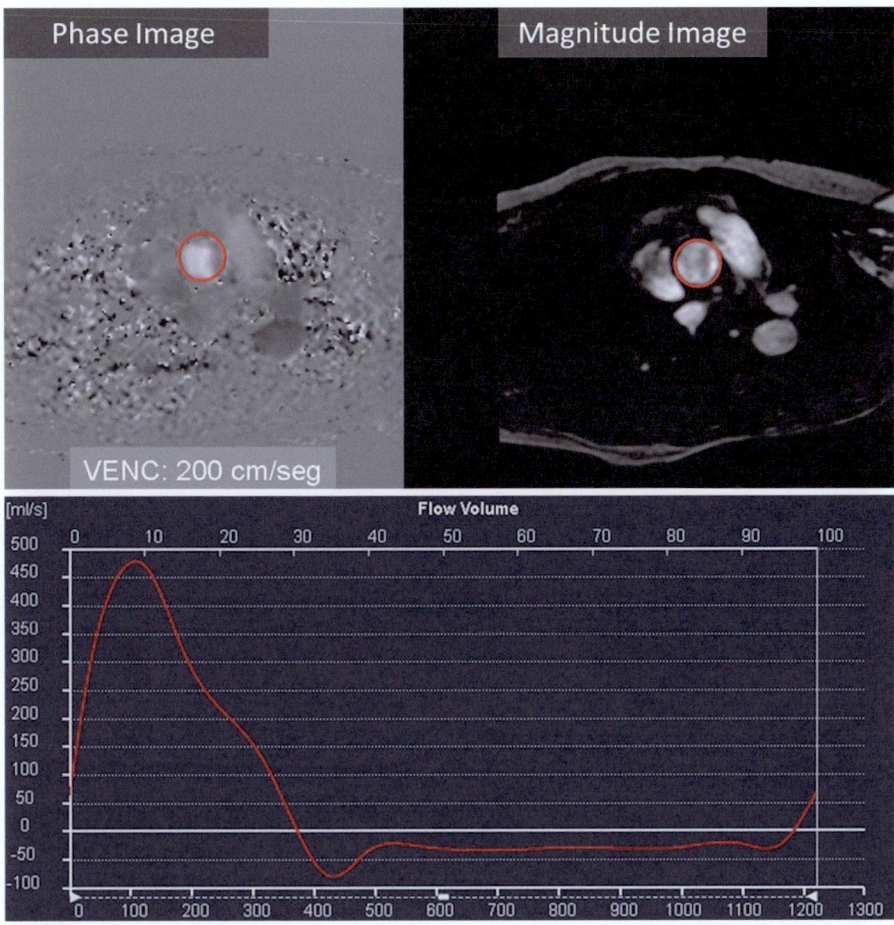

Fig. 7.14 (continued)

Recommended Bibliography

1. Bolen MA, Popovic ZB, Rajiah P, Gabriel RS, Zurick AO, Lieber ML et al (2011) Cardiac MR assessment of aortic regurgitation: holodiastolic flow reversal in the descending aorta helps stratify severity. Radiology 260:98–104
2. Cawley PJ, Maki JH, Otto CM (2009) Cardiovascular magnetic resonance imaging for valvular heart disease: technique and validation. Circulation 119:468–478
3. Chan KMJ, Wage R, Symmonds K, Rahman-Haley S, Mohiaddin RH, Firmin DN et al (2008) Towards comprehensive assessment of mitral regurgitation using cardiovascular magnetic resonance. J Cardiovasc Magn Reson 10:61
4. Gabriel RS, Renapurkar R, Bolen MA, Verhaert D, Leiber M, Flamm SD et al (2011) Comparison of severity of aortic regurgitation by cardiovascular magnetic resonance versus transthoracic echocardiography. Am J Cardiol 108:1014–1020
5. Myerson SG (2012) Heart valve disease: investigation by cardiovascular magnetic resonance. J Cardiovasc Magn Reson 14:7

CMR Study Protocols for Congenital Heart Diseases

Alberto Hidalgo

8.1 Introduction

Over recent decades there have been advances in paediatric cardiology and cardiac surgery that have allowed a significant number of patients with congenital heart disease (CHD) to live until adulthood. A proportion of these patients undergo palliative surgery in the first years of their lives which will require follow-up studies by imaging techniques to optimise treatment and plan further surgical procedures. Echocardiography is at the forefront of the diagnostic process in CHD, although cardiovascular magnetic resonance (CMR) has emerged as a technique that, due to its versatility and multiple diagnostic possibilities, provides with useful information on most relevant aspects of the diagnostic workup in these patients and is increasingly required in these patients. As with any other technique, CMR has also some limitations, but, fortunately, recent developments in multi-detector row computed tomography (MDCT) have made possible the addition of this technique to the array of imaging diagnostic resources for the management of patients with CHD.

Some of the advantages of CMR are particularly relevant in the field of CHD. CMR is a standard technique due to its reliability and reproducibility in the measurement of the volume and function of the cardiac chambers, particularly the right ventricle, which is hard to analyse by other techniques. This information is essential in patients with CHD, because many clinical decisions are based on changes of right ventricular volume or ejection fraction that occur over time, rather than on absolute values. The absence of ionising radiation is also particularly convenient, as these patients will probably be submitted to repeat examinations throughout their lives. Although transthoracic echocardiography is quite appropriate in newborn children, in adult patients ultrasound has some limitations, given its

---

A. Hidalgo, MD, PhD
Cardiac Imaging Unit, Radiology Department, Hospital de la Santa Creu i Sant Pau,
Universitat Autònoma de Barcelona, Barcelona, Spain
e-mail: JHidalgoP@santpau.cat

reduced field of view and suboptimal acoustic windows, particularly in those with a history of prior surgery. CMR, on the other hand, has the advantage of a wide field of view and multiplane imaging, which is fundamental for studying anatomical relations among both intracardiac and extracardiac structures.

Limitations of CMR in patients with CHD are due, mainly, to interferences in the images due to the presence of arrhythmias and artefacts resulting from respiratory movements. There may also be susceptibility artefacts in the images caused by metallic stents or prosthetic valves, although none of these conditions constitute a contraindication for the performance of a CMR study.

The study of patients with CHD benefits from all sequences with cardiac applications discussed in Chap. 1, although some of them are of particular interest in this setting. (1) "Black blood" TSE sequences, for instance, are useful for a morphological study that includes the anatomical relations between structures, which is in many cases are complex, and this helps in planning additional sequences. (2) Balanced TFE cine sequences are used in the conventional anatomical planes (2-chamber, 4-chamber and short axis), although in some cases may be necessary to perform additional specific sequences depending on the particular disease. (3) Phase-contrast sequences are used for studying the direction, velocity and volume of flow within native vessels or surgical graft conduits, which is essential in the assessment of valvular stenosis or regurgitation and, particularly, for the calculation of the pulmonary-to-systemic flow ratio (Qp/Qs), which defines the significance of intra- or extracardiac abnormal shunts. (4) Finally, MR contrast angiography is used when detailed anatomical information about the thoracic vessels is required, which is important in the assessment of the size and distribution of the pulmonary artery and its branches, or for the visualisation of aortopulmonary collateral circulation.

8.2 Sequential Segmental Analysis for the CMR Study of CHD

Sequential segmental analysis of the cardiac anatomy allows us to identify and properly classify the type of CHD in a comprehensible manner. The three anatomical segments that must be described by a systematic approach are the visceroatrial *situs*, the atrioventricular connection and the position and connections of the great vessels.

8.2.1 Determination of the Visceroatrial Situs

There are three possible types of *situs*: *solitus* (S,-,-), *inversus* (I,-,-) or ambiguous (A,-,-). The type of the *situs* is defined by the position of the atria and the adjacent organs. This requires a proper identification of the right and left atria. The right atrium has an appendage which is wide and triangular in shape, while the left atrium has a narrow, elongated, finger-like appendage. When the identification of the atria is uncertain, the position of other organs, such as the bronchial tree and the pulmonary artery, and the location of the liver, stomach and

8 CMR Study Protocols for Congenital Heart Diseases

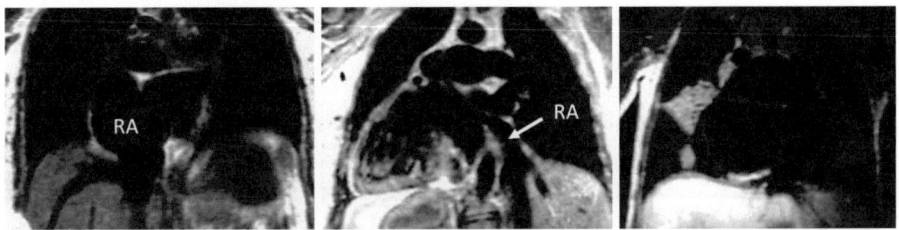

Fig. 8.1 Black blood T1w SE sequences in coronal plane showing the position of the right atrium (*RA*) in *situs solitus* (*left panel*) and *situs inversus* (*centre panel*), while in *situs* ambiguous (*right panel*), there is no clear distinction between right and left atria

spleen may help to define the *situs*. In *situs solitus*, the normal configuration, the right atrium and the liver are found at the right side, and the left atrium, stomach and spleen at the left (see Fig. 8.1, left panel). There is also a right lung with three lobes and a left one with two, the right pulmonary artery being located at the level of the main right one bronchus (eparterial bronchus), while the left pulmonary artery lies above the main left bronchus (hyparterial bronchus). In *situs inversus*, the anatomical configuration is the opposite of that in *situs solitus* (see Fig. 8.1, central panel). When the *situs* is neither *solitus* nor *inversus*, we speak of *situs* ambiguous or heterotaxy syndrome (see Fig. 8.1, right panel). *Situs* ambiguous frequently associates extracardiac malformations (splenic anomalies, biliary atresia and intestinal malrotation), as well as other cardiac anomalies.

8.2.2 Determination of the Atrioventricular Connection

Cardiovascular structures develop embryologically from a primitive cardiac tube that, during its evolution, will normally rotate rightward forming a D-loop (-,D,-) or, instead, abnormally, towards the left, in an L-loop (-,L,-). This determines the relations between the atria and the ventricles. Important for the study of atrioventricular connections is the identification of the anatomical right and left ventricles. The morphologically right ventricle is recognised by its triangular shape, trabeculated walls and by the presence of the moderator band (see arrow in Fig. 8.2, left panel). The morphologically left ventricle has smoother walls. Also, the papillary muscles in the right ventricle are located in the free wall and in the septum (see arrow, in Fig. 8.3), while in the left ventricle they are only found in the free wall. It is also helpful to identify the tricuspid and mitral valves, as the mitral is always part of the anatomically left ventricle and the tricuspid of the right one; the tricuspid valve is characterised by a septal insertion of its valvular ring displaced towards the apex of the heart in relation to the mitral annulus (see arrow in Fig. 8.4). When the morphologically right atrium connects with the morphologically right ventricle, there is atrioventricular concordance; when it does not, there is atrioventricular discordance (see Fig. 8.4).

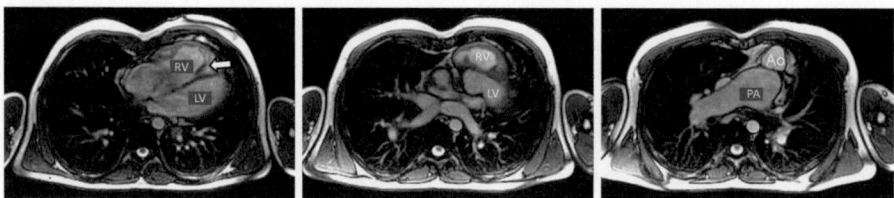

Fig. 8.2 Frames from SSFP cine sequences oriented on strict transverse planes used for a segmental analysis of the cardiac structures (see text for explanation). The right ventricle (*RV*) is identified by the presence of the moderator band (*arrow*, in *left panel*) and is shown to be connected to the aorta (*Ao*), while the left ventricle (*LV*) connects with the pulmonary artery (*PA*), corresponding thus the case to a transposition of the great arteries

Fig. 8.3 Frame from an SSFP sequence in short axis where the right ventricle (*RV*) is identified by the presence of a papillary muscle in a position adjacent to the interventricular septum (*arrow*)

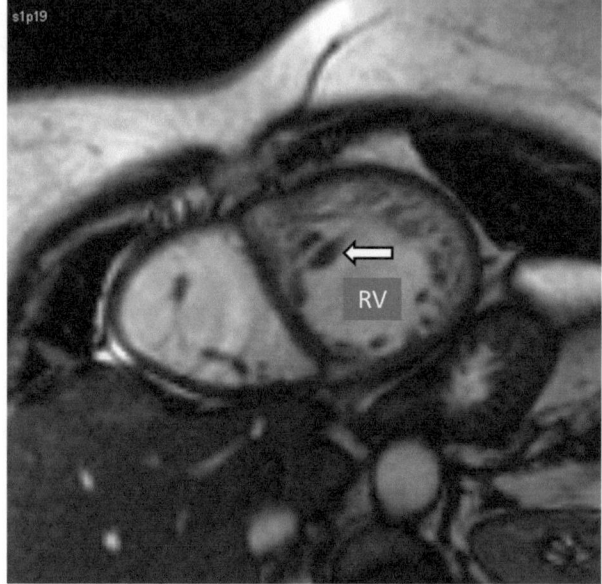

8.2.3 Determination of the Origin and Position of the Great Vessels

The aorta and the pulmonary artery may be in normal position (*solitus*) (-,-,S), in inverted position (-,-,I), in D-transposition (-,-,DTGV), in L-transposition (-,-,LTGV), in D-malposition (-,-,DMGV) or in L-malposition (-,-,LMGV). The term "malposition" refers to that situation where it is impossible to determine in which ventricle the large vessels originate or, also, when the vessels emerge from a single ventricle. The term "transposition" is used when the aorta emerges from the right ventricle and the pulmonary artery from the left one. There are two types of transposition: D-transposition (S,D,DTGV) and L-transposition (S,L,LTGV). In D-transposition, atrioventricular concordance

Fig. 8.4 Frame from an SSFP sequence in four-chamber view where the tricuspid valve (*arrow*) is identified by its more apical position in relation with the mitral valve. Despite of being connected to the left atrium (*LA*), the triscupid valve is always part of an anatomical right ventricle (*RV*), an observation that permits, in this case, a diagnosis of ventricular inversion to be made

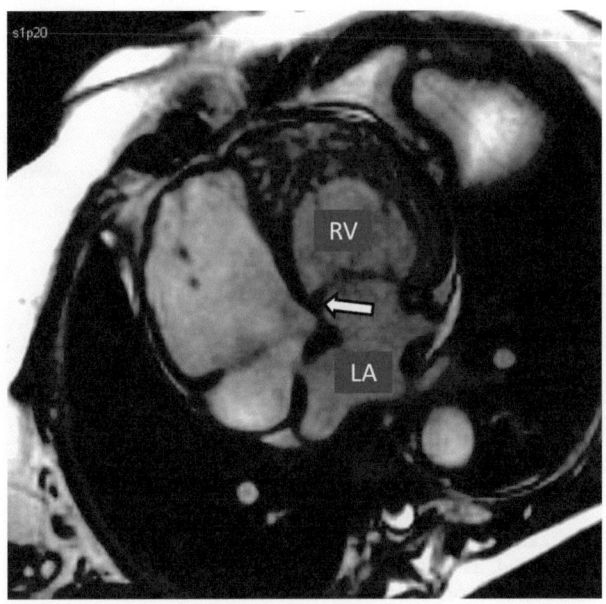

is normal, but the aorta is located anterior to the pulmonary artery and emerges from the right ventricle (see Fig. 8.2, middle and right panels). In L-transposition, the relationship between the large vessels and the ventricles is inverted, but because there is no atrioventricular concordance (L-loop), the circulation is "corrected" (corrected transposition of the great vessels or double discordance) (see Fig. 8.5).

8.3 Assessment of the Origin of the Coronary Arteries

An anomalous origin of one or more coronary arteries from the sinuses of Valsalva is not a rare anomaly, as it is present in nearly 1 % of the population either as an isolate finding or in association with other congenital defects. The potential for clinical symptoms is variable, but patients with some particular forms are definitely at risk of sudden death. CMR, by means of the whole heart coronary MRA sequence, is adequate for identifying the origin of the coronary vessels from the aortic root and their proximal course, this allowing the detection of anomalous anatomical patterns (see Fig. 8.6).

Although MDCT has advantages for the study of the coronary arteries, the assessment of the origin of the vessels by MRA is feasible as a part of a comprehensive CMR exam to rule out some structural background for sudden death.

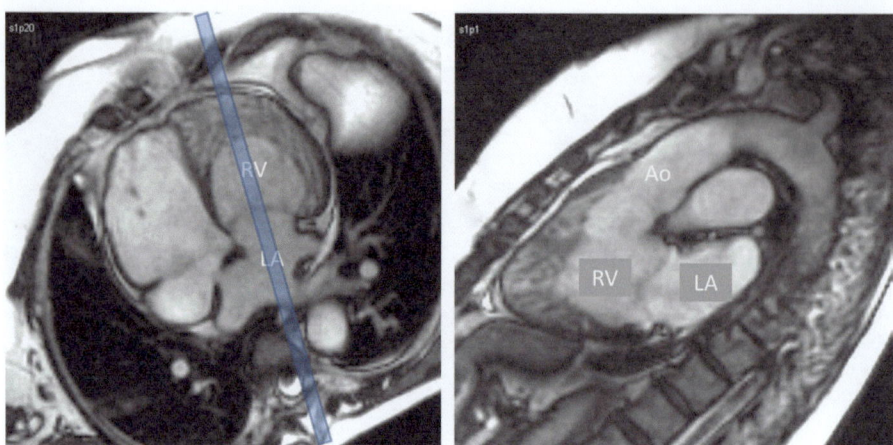

Fig. 8.5 Planning of an SSFP cine slice on the plane shown in Fig. 8.4 (*left panel*) with a vertical longitudinal orientation on the right ventricle (*RV*). The resultant plane (*right panel*) shows that the vessel arising from the RV is the aorta (*Ao*). As the blood flowing through the aorta is, in fact, oxygenated, as it comes from the left atrium (*LA*), via the RV, this malformation is called "corrected" transposition of the great vessels

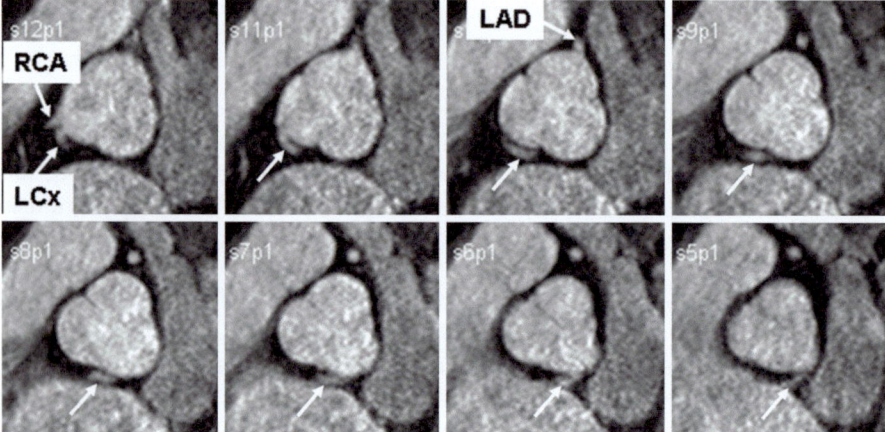

Fig. 8.6 Slices form a whole heart MRA sequence oriented on the aortic root for the study of the origin of the coronary arteries. An abnormal origin is seen of the left circumflex artery (LCx) from the right sinus of Valsalva, independent from the right coronary artery (*RCA*), while the left anterior descending (LAD) arises from the left coronary sinus. From its origin, the LCx follows a course between the aortic root and both atria (*unlabeled arrows*) towards its normal position at the left lateral aspect of the heart

8.4 Use of CMR in the Most Frequent Types of CHD

8.4.1 Intracardiac and Extracardiac Shunts

Interatrial and interventricular septal defects and the patency of the *ductus arteriosus* are the most common non-cyanotic CHD. They cause a left-right shunting of blood that leads to a volume overload of the cardiac chambers, the significance of which depends on the size of the defect. The CMR study is aimed, in these cases, to the following objectives:

- *Evaluation of ventricular volumes.* An essential part of the study of shunts is the assessment of their effect upon the right and/or the left ventricular volumes, depending on their location. The study protocol for ventricular volume and function described in Chap. 1 is applied.
- *Visualisation of the defect.* Balanced TFE cine sequences oriented according to the specific defect to be studied are appropriate. For atrial septal defect of the *ostium secundum* type, cine sequences in 4-chamber orientation are useful (see Fig. 8.7, arrows), but we also recommend a series of multiple cine slices oriented orthogonally to the axis of the aortic root (see Fig. 8.8 left panel), which allows a scan of the whole interatrial septum, where we can detect the defect and, also, to visualise a signal void of the flow shunted through it into the right atrium (see Fig. 8.8, arrows in the right panel). The complete study of the interatrial septum with this strategy allows the detection of defects at peripheral regions of the septum, such as those of venous sinus type (see Fig. 8.9, arrow).

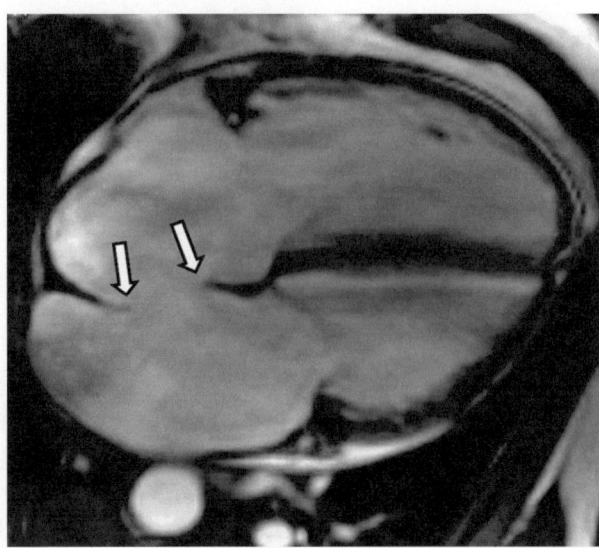

Fig. 8.7 Frame from an SSFP sequence in four-chamber view where the presence of a large atrial septal defect of the *ostium secundum* type is detected (*arrows*)

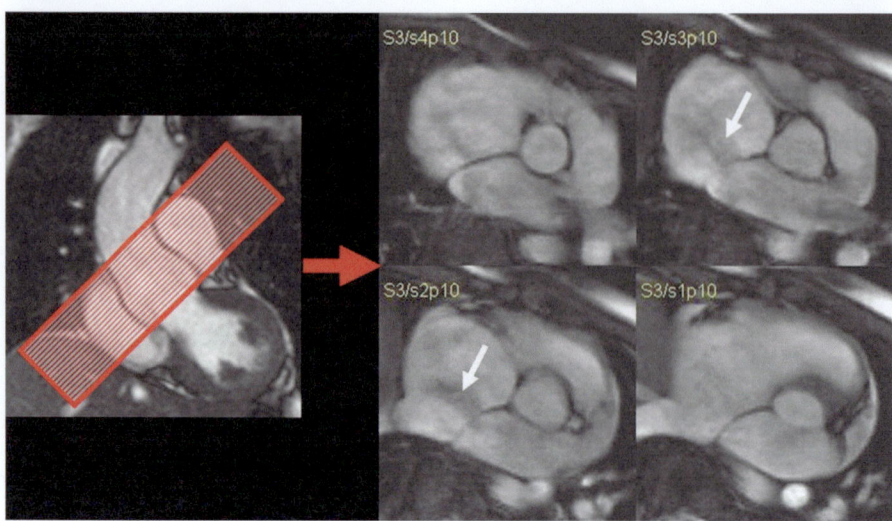

Fig. 8.8 Planning of a series of SSFP cine sequences on a coronal localizer plane with an orthogonal orientation to the longitudinal axis of the aortic root (*stack of red lines, left panel*). The resultant cine slices (*right panels*) permit, in case of an atrial septal defect of the *ostium secundum* type, to detect the size and position of the defect and, also, to visualise the signal void caused by the flow through it (*white arrows*)

Fig. 8.9 Frame from an SSFP sequence oriented on the atria showing the presence of a septal defect of the *sinus venosus* type located at the junction of the right atrium and the superior vena cava (*arrow*)

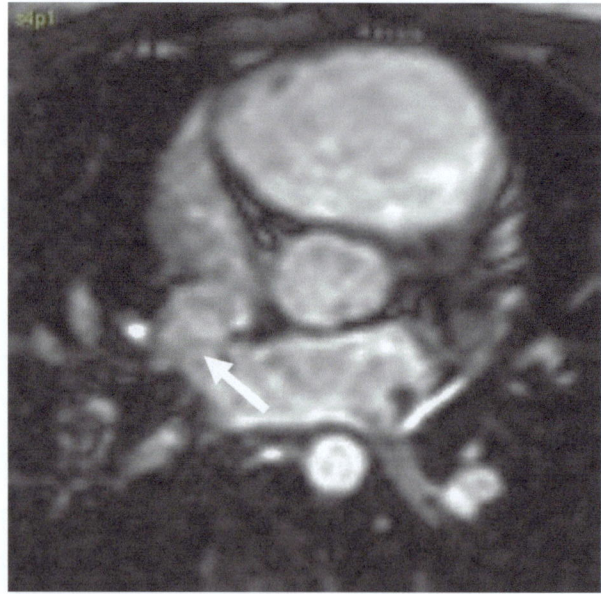

Ventricular septal defects require multiple cine sequences in 4-chamber orientation (see Fig. 8.10, arrow in the left panel), which may be complemented by short-axis slices oriented on the defect (see Fig. 8.10, right panel). Once again, visualisation

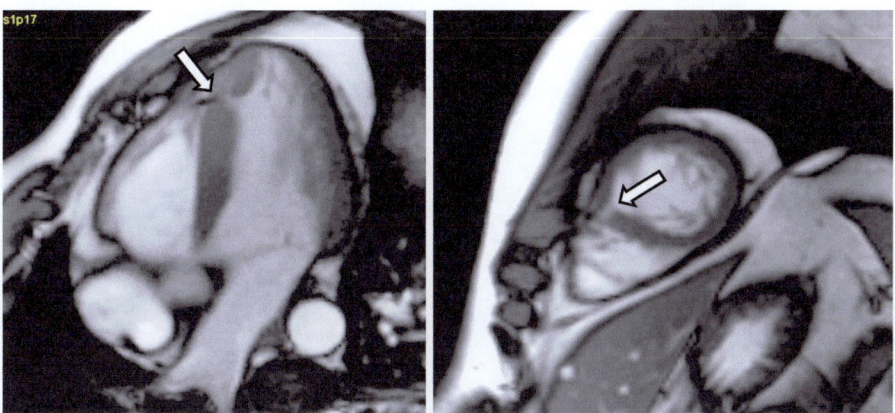

Fig. 8.10 Frames from SSFP cine sequences oriented on longitudinal and short-axis planes showing a ventricular septal defect of the muscular type (*arrows*)

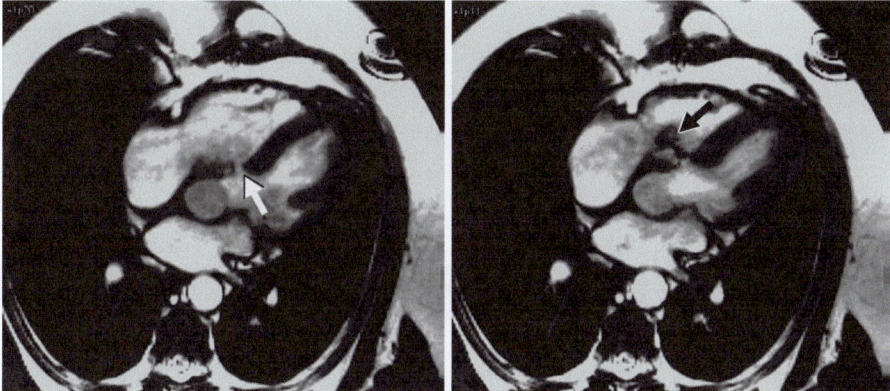

Fig. 8.11 Diastolic (*left panel*) and systolic (*right panel*) frames from an SSFP cine sequence showing a membranous ventricular septal defect (*white arrow*) and the signal void due to turbulent flow through it (*black arrow*)

of the flow turbulence through the defect helps in its localisation (see Fig. 8.11, arrow in the right panel).

The study of a patent *ductus arteriosus* requires an MR contrast angiography, although, in cases of a vessel with a certain diameter, it is possible to visualise it in cine sequences oriented on the plane of the aorta (see Fig. 8.12, arrow).

- *Calculation of the Qp/Qs ratio.* The study is performed with phase-contrast sequences oriented along orthogonal planes of the ascending aorta and the main pulmonary artery (see Chap. 1, Figs. 1.24 and 1.25). In case of an intracardiac left-to-right shunt, the flow volume at the pulmonary artery is increased with respect to the one at the aorta in proportion with the amount of the shunt. The Qp/

Fig. 8.12 Frame from an SSFP sequence oriented on the plane of a patent *ductus arteriosus* (*arrow*) communicating the inferior aspect of the aortic arch (*Ao*) with a fairly enlarged pulmonary artery (*PA*)

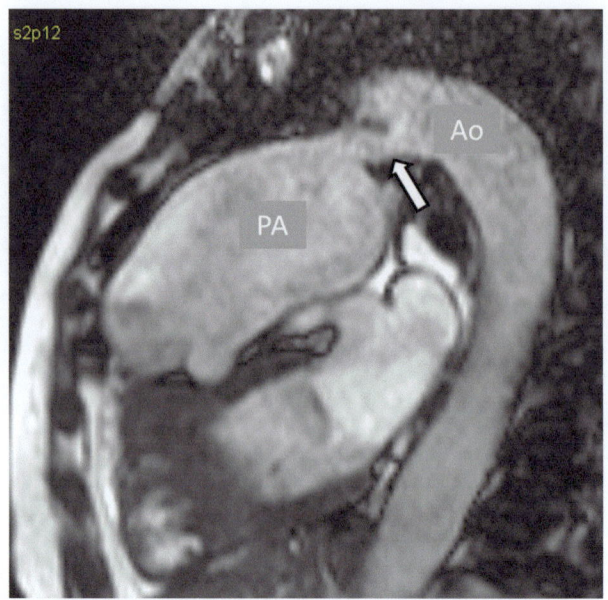

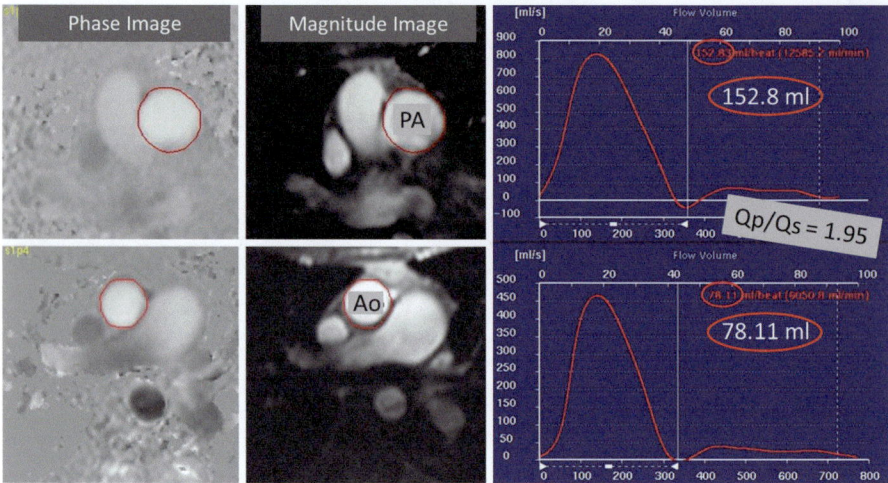

Fig. 8.13 Method for calculating the pulmonary-to-systemic flow ratio (*Qp/Qs*) by CMR. Phase-contrast sequences are obtained from cross-sectional planes of the pulmonary artery (*PA*) and the ascending aorta (*Ao*) (*left panels*): the quotient between the pulmonary and aortic systolic volumes derived from the flow curves (*right panels*) corresponds to the Qp/Qs ratio

Qs ratio expresses thus the overload of the pulmonary circulation due to the defect and may be used to quantify its significance. The calculation of this ratio by CMR is particularly reliable, the technique being considered as a standard of reference for this purpose (see Fig. 8.13).

8.4.2 Tetralogy of Fallot (T4F)

Tetralogy of Fallot is the most frequent cyanotic CHD (nearly 10% of the whole group). The four components of the anomaly are pulmonary stenosis (subvalvular), ventricular septal defect, overriding of the aorta upon the defect, and hypertrophy of the right ventricle. The current indication, in adult patients with T4F, is the assessment of heart function after surgical repair, which is usually performed at infancy. Objectives of a CMR study in these patients are:

- *Assessment of pulmonary valve function.* Anatomical correction of T4F frequently results in some degree of residual pulmonary valve regurgitation, which may be significant in a proportion of patients. Phase-contrast sequences oriented along the main pulmonary artery allow the volume and regurgitant fraction of the pulmonary valve to be determined (see Chap. 7, Fig. 7.11). CMR has become a standard of reference for this calculation, which is important for the management of these patients.
- *Evaluation of right ventricular volume and function.* When the degree of pulmonary regurgitation is more than moderate, the volume overload of the right ventricle may be prominent and lead to dilatation and reduced systolic function of the chamber (see Fig. 8.14). Serial measurements of these parameters are important because progressive impairment of right ventricular function may lead to an indication for pulmonary valve replacement in these patients. Regional dyskinesia or aneurysmal areas of the right ventricular outflow tract are also potential complications of surgery that can be assessed by the CMR study.

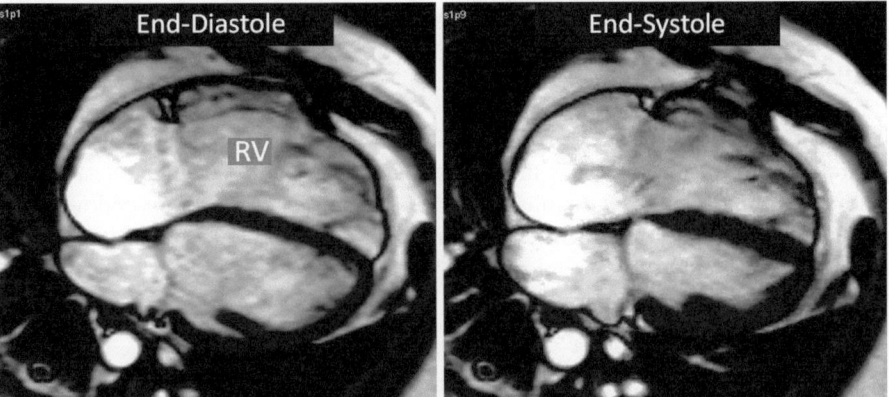

Fig. 8.14 End-diastolic (*left panel*) and end-systolic (*right panel*) frames from an SSFP cine sequence on four-chamber view in a case of operated tetralogy of Fallot with significant pulmonary regurgitation: note the marked enlargement of the right ventricle (*RV*) and its reduced contractile function

- *Recognition of other complications.* Although a residual intracardiac shunt after intervention is rare, a CMR study can definitely rule it out by calculating the Qp/Qs ratio. Tricuspid insufficiency is generally due to right ventricular dilation. Its quantification, though less reliable than that of pulmonary insufficiency, can be performed with a combination of right ventricular volume and pulmonary flow (see Chap. 7). Other potential complications to be assessed by the CMR study include dilation of the aortic root and residual aortic regurgitation after repair of the septal defect.

8.4.3 Coarctation of the Aorta

Coarctation of the aorta is appropriately studied by MDCT that provides unique anatomical information on the anomaly, including the presence and extent of collateral circulation. CMR, however, is also relevant as it allows the grading of the obstruction and its functional consequences. Again, the CMR study is usually required in the follow-up of patients submitted to surgical repair. CMR is useful then in two aspects:

Assessment of the Degree of Stenosis or Restenosis After Surgery
Phase-contrast flow sequences may be performed with an orthogonal orientation to the aorta distally to the site of coarctation for the measurement of the maximal flow velocity and, thus, the pressure gradient through the stenosis. The magnitude of collateral flow may also be calculated by determining the volume flow at the descending aorta immediately after the coarctation (see Fig. 8.15, upper panel) and also at the level of the diaphragmatic aorta (see Fig. 8.15, middle panel). Any increase in volume flow from these proximal to distal sample sites is due to re-entry of flow to the descending aorta from collateral circulation developed to bypass the coarctation (see Fig. 8.15, lower panel). A contrast MR angiography also permits to visualise the collateral circulation, by any of its modes of presentation, either 3D rendering or MIP (see Fig. 8.16).

Study of Complications from Previous Surgery The surgical treatment of aortic coarctation frequently includes the performance of termino-terminal anastomoses with resection of the aortic segments or the use of prosthetic tubes or endovascular stents. These techniques may be complicated at long term by the formation of local

Fig. 8.15 Method for calculating the amount of collateral flow in cases of aortic coarctation. Phase-contrast sequences are performed at the level of the descending aorta immediately distal to the stenosis (*red line, upper left panel*) and, also, at the diaphragmatic segment of the vessel (*white line, middle panel*). Differences in flow volume at these levels (*lower panel*) are proportional to the amount of collateral flow bypassing the coarctation

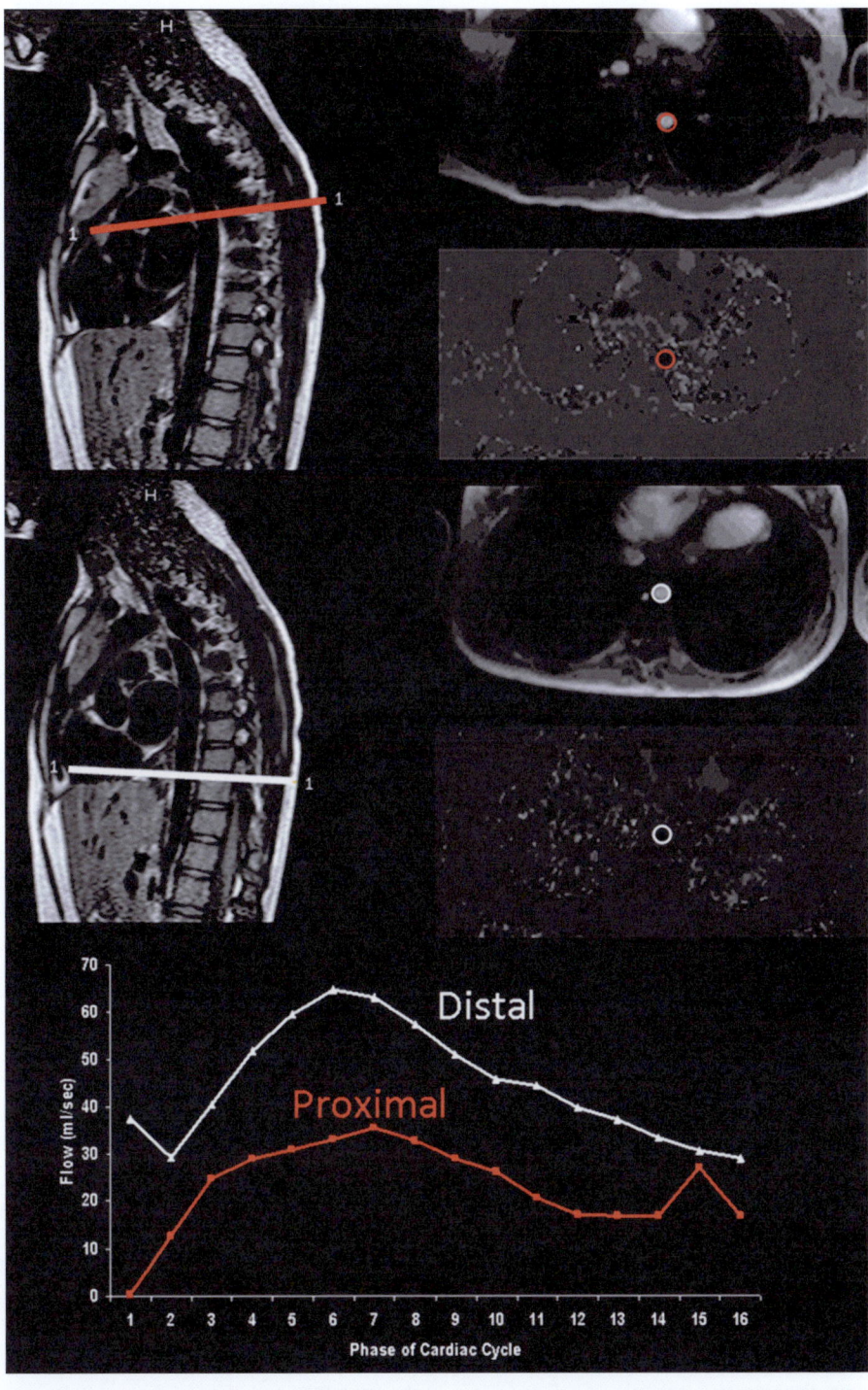

Fig. 8.16 MIP reconstruction of an MR contrast angiography of the aorta in a case of coarctation. The location and morphology of the involved segment is shown (*black arrow*) as well as an extensive network of collateral circulation (*white arrows*)

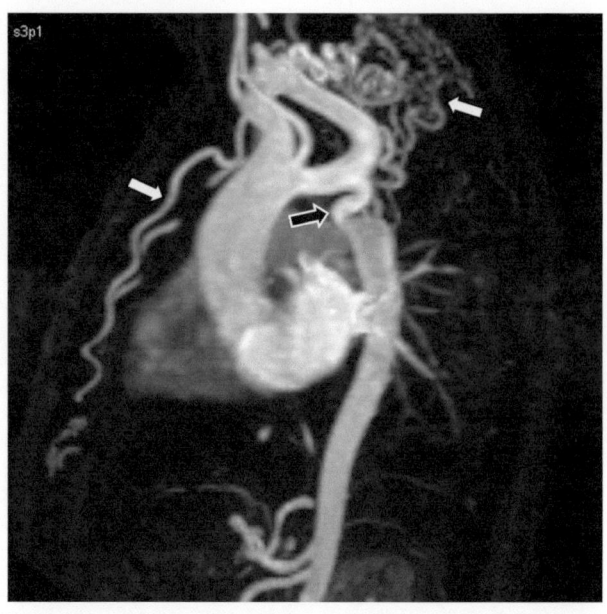

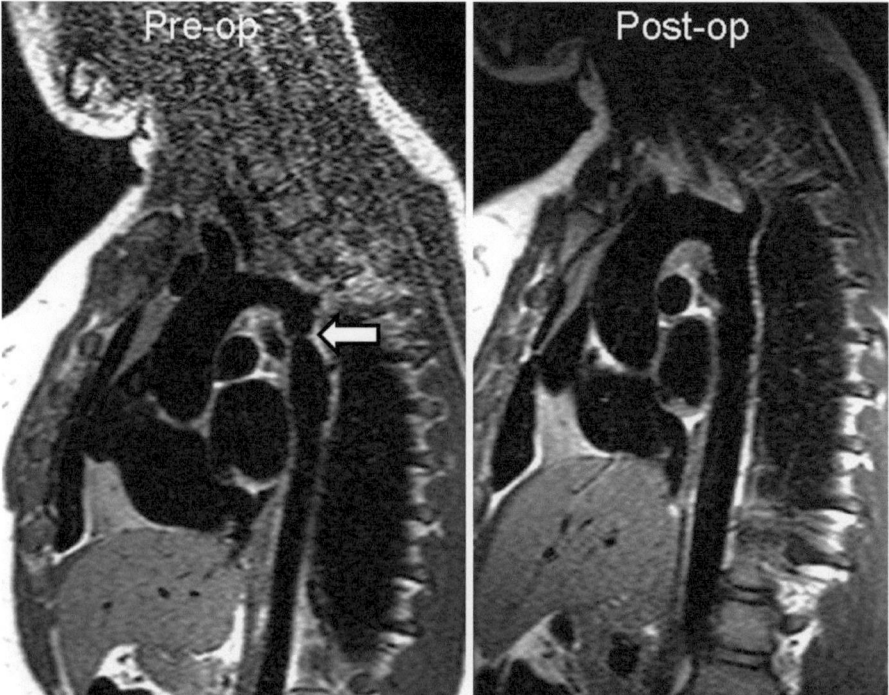

Fig. 8.17 Black blood T1w SE sequences oriented on the plane of the thoracic aorta in a patient with diaphragmatic coarctation before (*arrow*, in the *left panel*) and after (*right panel*) surgical correction

aneurysms or recoarctation. For this reason, a CMR study performed after the operation (see Fig. 8.17) is useful as a reference for these complications to be appropriately identified during the follow-up.

Recommended Bibliography

1. Kilner PJ, Geva T, Kaemmerer H, Trindade PT, Schwitter J, Webb GD (2010) Recommendations for cardiovascular magnetic resonance in adults with congenital heart disease from the respective working groups of the European Society of Cardiology. Eur Heart J 31:794–805
2. Lapierre C, Déry J, Guérin R, Viremouneix L, Dubois J, Garel L (2010) Segmental approach to imaging of congenital heart disease. Radiographics 30:397–411
3. Rajiah P, Kanne JP (2011) Cardiac MRI: part 1. Cardiovascular shunts. AJR Am J Roentgenol 197:W603–W620

Protocols for Cardiac Studies with Computed Tomography

9

Rubén Leta and Antonio Barros

9.1 Introduction

Cardiac computed tomography (CCT) is a radiological technique that provides information on the cardiac and thoracic anatomy. The technological development of the equipment, in the late 1990s and early 2000s, which permits submillimetric slices of the cardiac structures to be acquired, has allowed the application of this examination in the analysis of the coronary anatomy.

Before these technological advances, cardiac studies were already performed – by CT with electron emission – to evaluate the presence and degree of coronary wall calcification. However, it was not until the early 2000s when multidetector systems, giving an adequate spatial resolution and wide anatomical coverage, allowed the acquirement of a reliable non-invasive coronary contrast angiography.

Today's CT equipment is able to perform any kind of study of the heart and related structures (e.g. pericardium, aorta, pulmonary arteries and veins). Nevertheless, the following discussion will focus on non-invasive coronary angiography by CCT, in accordance with the recommendations of the Society of Cardiovascular Computed Tomography.

9.2 Equipment

The basic equipment required for the practice of a non-invasive coronary angiography consists of, at least, a 16-row multidetector CT (MDCT). Although coronary studies using 4-row systems have been reported, inadequate coverage of the axial axis (Z) with a reasonable spatial resolution limits their usefulness for coronary

R. Leta, MD, PhD (✉) • A. Barros, MD
Cardiac Imaging Unit, Cardiology Department, Hospital de la Santa Creu i Sant Pau,
Universitat Autònoma de Barcelona, Barcelona, Spain
e-mail: rleta@santpau.cat

angiography, although they may be used for the study of coronary calcium. On the other hand, even with 16-row equipment, a relatively high number of cardiac beats is needed to reconstruct images, which means a longer, more unstable breath hold, and the possibility of cardiac and respiratory motion artefacts.

In the space of a few years, the fast technological development in the field has produced MDCT systems with 32, 64, 256 and 320 rows of detectors as well as others with dual emission. This has drastically changed the former axial coverage limitation; nowadays acquiring a non-invasive coronary angiography is feasible in the interval of one or two heart beats, meaning a very short breath hold, which contributes to improved quality of the images acquired. Nevertheless, as the use of late-generation equipment for cardiac imaging is still not general, we may consider 64- row, single emission equipment to be the standard technology for CCT. These systems should permit rotation times <420 ms (ideally <350 ms), to obtain an adequate temporal resolution, while the detector thickness should be <0.75 mm, for an optimal spatial resolution. Obviously, a software appropriate for cardiac examinations, synchronised with the electrocardiogram (ECG), must be available. In its most basic form, these systems will perform a helical acquisition (continuous during several cardiac cycles) with retrospective reconstruction, with the possibility of performing the acquisition with dose modulation in order to reduce the total radiation of the exam being recommended.

In this chapter we will refer to a particular device (Philips Brilliance iCT), although the information provided is also applicable to other systems. This equipment allows 256 images to be obtained per rotation, at a rotational speed of 270 ms and with an axial coverage of 80 mm per rotation.

9.2.1 Radiation in Cardiac CT Studies

The radiation administered by MDCT devices has been the subject of great debate and depends on many factors: emission type (simple, double), gantry rotation, filters, voltage and intensity of current in the X-ray tube, amplitude and duration of the acquisition, slice thickness, pitch, type of acquisition, etc.

The type of acquisition is an important factor in the radiation dose. In helical acquisition with tube current modulation, the device reduces the current of the tube and, thus, the radiation, during most of the systolic phase of the cardiac cycle, a time period in which the coronary arteries are submitted to movement due to ventricular contraction, which makes the acquisition of the exam during this phase unreliable. In contrast, during diastole when the coronary arteries are less subjected to motion, the system automatically increases the tube current to provide the adequate level for the study. With this dose modulation, the radiation may be reduced by nearly 50 % without affecting the quality of the coronary imaging and, importantly, while still being able to acquire the information over the whole cardiac cycle, as images obtained at low dosage (in systole) can be reliably used to calculate ventricular volumes and function. A limitation of this modality is that it is only applicable if the heart rhythm is regular and the heart rate (HR) <65 beats per minute (bpm).

The technological advance of MDCT and the introduction of systems with a high number of row detectors have led to dramatic reductions in the acquisition time. In addition, the introduction of prospective acquisition (step and shoot) has allowed even a further reduction of the radiation dose, which, with today's equipment, is less than 80–90 % of that of conventional systems. In this type of acquisition, which is the optimal one when available, radiation is limited to a very short diastolic period of the cardiac cycle (within 70–80 % of the RR cycle), although it requires a regular cardiac rhythm with a HR <65 bpm. This mode of examination, on the other hand, does not allow the analysis of ventricular volumes and function, as the acquisition is limited to the mentioned time phase.

The importance of the tube voltage for the radiation dose, which is proportional to the square of the change in voltage, is well known. In recent studies, it has been shown that a reduction in the voltage of cardiac studies from 120 kV (the standard) to 100 kV in subjects with a weight <85 kg and a body mass index (BMI) <30 kg/m^2 (non-obese) permits a reduction of approximately 30 % of the dosage. For all this, although it is still necessary to use voltages of 140 kV for significantly obese individuals with the double aim of improving tissue penetration and reducing noise, this level of voltage should be restricted to this group of subjects.

Finally, it should be mentioned that the appearance of fourth-generation iterative reconstruction systems has meant a new and important step in the reduction of radiation. In all, the estimated dose of radiation for an MDCT coronary angiography may be up to 20 millisievert (mSv) for early systems without tube modulation or prospective acquisition, which is reduced to 1–5 mSv when these modalities are available. This dose of radiation compares favourably with that of an invasive diagnostic coronary angiography, which ranges between 2 and 20 mSv.

9.3 Preparation of the Patient

9.3.1 Pretest Assessment

An MDCT coronary angiography should be prescribed by medical staff with a basic knowledge of the benefits and potential risks associated with the examination. Contraindications include known previous anaphylactic reaction to iodinated contrast, inability to cooperate in the acquirement of the study (to remain quietly in a supine position on the examination table or to raise their arms), inability to perform a correct breath hold, pregnancy, clinically unstable condition (decompensated heart failure, hypotension or uncontrolled arrhythmia) and chronic renal insufficiency with glomerular filtration <30 ml/min in a non-dialysed patient.

At the time of ordering the exam, the patient must be adequately informed of its advantages and disadvantages and sign an informed written consent form. Likewise, precise instructions should be given prior to the examination, which include not ingesting solid food for up to 4 h prior to the study, although adequate hydration must be maintained, which is a recognised measure of renal protection from contrast.

9.3.2 Preparation of the Patient at the Time of the Examination

Preparation of the patient aims to achieve and maintain a regular stable heart rhythm, if possible with an HR <65 bpm (ideally <60 bpm), and an adequate breath hold. The patient's anthropometric variables should be noted (weight, size, body mass index) in order to adjust the parameters of the X-ray tube current and the volume of contrast. Patients with a BMI <30 can be subjected to a study with lower voltage (100 kV), which significantly reduces the effective radiation dose without deterioration of the image quality, while those with a BMI >40 are not considered ideal candidates for a coronary study by MDCT, given the poor image quality expected.

9.3.2.1 Premedication

Most MDCT systems provide higher image quality when the cardiac rhythm is stable, regular and slow (<65 bpm), which, in the appropriate equipment, allow for a prospective acquisition, with the consequent reduction of the radiation dose of the study. In this sense, the administration of beta-blockers remains crucial, metoprolol being the most widely used agent. It may be given orally (100 mg, 1 h before the study), though many groups prefer an intravenous administration of a dose of 5 mg immediately before performing the study, which is repeated at 5-min intervals if the appropriate HR is not achieved, with a maximum recommended dose of 15 mg. Metoprolol is contraindicated in the case of allergy, active bronchospasm or decompensated heart failure; in these cases the use of alternative agents, such as diltiazem or oral ivabradine, is favoured.

In the absence of contraindications, the administration of nitrates prior to a coronary MDCT study leads to vasodilation which translates to improved image quality, especially if the patient also receives the beta-blocker agent to abolish the possible reflex tachycardia induced by nitrates. The recommended dose is of 400–800 μg (one to two tablets) sublingually, 5–10 min before image acquisition. Blood pressure monitoring is necessary in these cases.

9.3.2.2 Administration of Contrast

A coronary MDCT exam is, in fact, a non-invasive angiographic study and, as such, requires contrast to be administered to enhance the coronary vascular tree. A study of optimal quality requires an intra-arterial level of radiodensity of, at least, 250 Hounsfield units (HU) (in practice >350 HU, in proximal coronary segments).

In non-allergic patients, iodinated contrast is used in a concentration of between 300 and 350 mg/ml. In coronary MDCT studies, administration through an injection pump that permits a flow >5 ml/s (usually 5–6 ml/s) is recommended, with a double-head system that allows flushing with saline solution (40–50 cm^3) after the administration of contrast. This is administered by intravenous injection into a peripheral vein, ideally the right antecubital vein, because a large venous diameter is required to support a high flow of injection, which must always be performed with an 18–20 calibre cannula. The total volume of contrast to be given oscillates between 60 and 120 ml (1 ml/kg, in adults), depending on the infusion velocity and the duration of the injection. The duration of the infusion should be at least equal or slightly superior to the estimated duration of the acquisition, although in acquisitions of short duration the infusion should be <10 s.

The synchronisation of the image acquisition with the arrival of the contrast in the anatomical structures for study is essential for obtaining a good quality study with adequate contrast throughout the whole acquisition. This can be done by using bolus test or bolus-tracking techniques. In the bolus test technique, a small amount of contrast is given (10–20 ml) followed by 50 ml of saline solution, and images are acquired of the ascending aorta every 1 or 2 s to assess the time at which an adequate density is achieved. In the bolus-tracking technique, a region of interest is placed on the ascending aorta (in 64-row systems) or the descending portion of the vessel (in 256–320-row devices), and images are acquired every 2 s after the start of the administration of the bolus. The system then automatically calculates the attenuation value (HU) in the region of interest and, when a predefined value is reached (normally between 140 and 180 HU), the patient is asked to start a breath hold and soon afterwards the whole acquisition is performed.

In the case of allergy to iodinated contrast agents, the study can reasonably be performed by using a 1 molar paramagnetic contrast agent (gadolinium compound), at a dose of 0.4 mmol/kg, without exceeding 50–60 ml in order to avoid nephrotoxicity.

9.4　Cardiac CT Protocols

All cardiac CT studies begin with a topogram (similar to a chest X-ray) (see Fig. 9.1), which is used to fix the acquisition limits of every study.

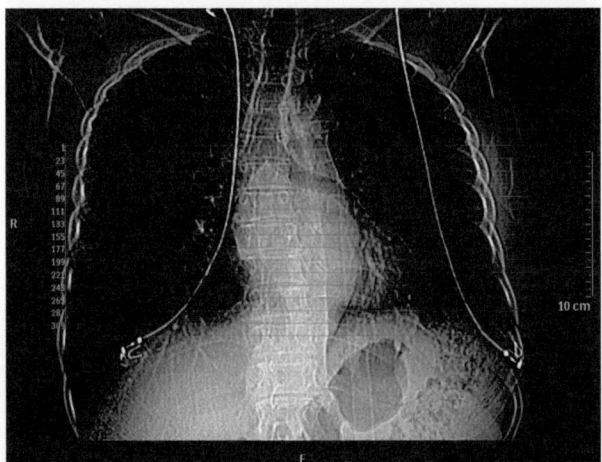

Fig. 9.1 Topogram for planning of the acquisition of a cardiac CT study

9.4.1 Coronary Calcium Study

This is the simplest of all cardiac CT examinations, as contrast is not needed and the radiation dose is low. It is highly sensitive in order to detect even minimal amounts of calcium in the coronary arterial wall, and its clinical value has been particularly shown in the screening of coronary risk factors:

- *Type of acquisition*: prospective in apnea, craniocaudal, from the carina of the trachea to the upper third of the abdomen.
- *RX tube parameters*: 120 kV, 210 mAs (effective mAs).
- *Acquisition period*: 75 % of RR interval.
- Contrast: no.
- Slice thickness: 3 mm.
- Reconstruction interval: 3 mm.
- *Reconstruction matrix*: 512 × 512 with hard filter.
- *Analysis*: specialised cardiac CT workstation software with measurement in all the slices of the area and density of all the zones identified as coronary calcium (>130 UH), calculation of volume and mass of calcium and conversion to Agatston units (see Fig. 9.2).
- *Report*: must include the total value of the Agatston score and the population percentile of the patient, taking into account their age and sex. Additionally, the score may be reported for every main coronary artery.

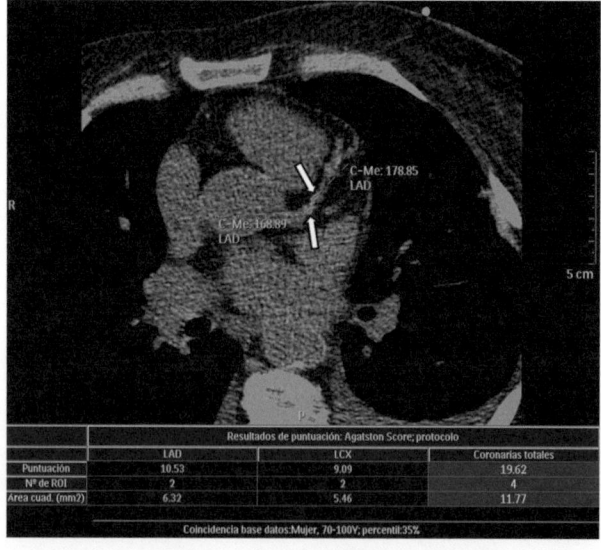

Fig. 9.2 Software analysis for detection of coronary artery calcium (*arrows*) and its conversion into Agatston units

9.4.2 Non-invasive Coronary Angiography

- Acquisition: apnea, craniocaudal, from the carina of trachea to the upper third of the abdomen. The mode of acquisition will depend on the rhythm and the HR:
  - Stable sinus rhythm with HR <65 bpm: prospective in apnea, craniocaudal, from the carina to the upper third of the abdomen. If there is no mode of prospective acquisition available in the system, alternatively, a helical acquisition with tube current modulation can be performed.
  - Irregular rhythm or HR >65 bpm (or HR <65 bpm but unstable): helical without tube current modulation.
- *RX tube parameters*: 100–120 kV (> 85 kg, BMI >30), 220–400 mAs.
- Acquisition process:
  - Prospective acquisition: 75% RR.
  - Helical acquisition: the whole cardiac cycle, with retrospective reconstruction every 5% of the RR (multiphase). The optimal phases for coronary analysis are usually found between 70 and 80% of the RR if the HR is <65 bpm and between 40 and 50% of the RR if the HR is >70 bpm. In the case of irregular rhythm (atrial fibrillation), the phase of 90% of the RR should also be considered suitable.
  - Finally, one of the two reconstruction modalities must be chosen: a half-scan (half a rotation) or segmental reconstruction. In the half-scan modality – the first choice if the HR is <65 bpm – the image is built up on the basis of the information obtained during one half of the gantry rotation, in a single cardiac cycle. In the segmental or multicycle reconstruction, the necessary information (half of the gantry rotation in single emission systems) is segmented and is acquired based on two or three cardiac cycles. This image will have better temporal resolution, especially in the case of high HR, but requires a perfectly regular cardiac rhythm and that the position of the heart does not change in the acquired beats.
- Contrast: iodine, intravenously, 60–120 ml at a speed of 5–6 ml/s. In the case of iodine allergy, a pretest desensitisation treatment should be prescribed, or, alternatively, 1 M gadolinium can be used (at a dose <60 ml).
- Slice thickness: always 1 mm (ideally <0.75 mm). Thicker slices add less noise to the image but have lower spatial resolution than thin slices.
- *Reconstruction interval*: 0.25–0.3 mm (50% of slice thickness).
- *Reconstruction matrix*: attempts must be made to accommodate the spatial resolution of the MDCT study with the resolution in pixels of the reconstructed image. For a field of view of 20–25 cm, a 512 × 512 matrix is recommended. Using larger fields of view will reduce the resolution.
- *Reconstruction filters* (*kernels*): these filters refer to the mathematical algorithms that compute the CT values (the raw data) in pixel values. Each manufacturer of MDCT equipment has their own filters, but they are all similar. It is recommended to use "intermediate" filters in most studies; "soft" filters for noisy images, particularly in obese patients; and "hard" filters with high resolution to reduce the effect of metals (stents) or calcium.
- *Analysis*: it is fundamental to check the images immediately after acquisition, as well as the ECG recordings, in the main console of the MDCT, before the patient

leaves the examination table. This permits the quality of the study to be evaluated and repeated if necessary. Also, if the MDCT equipment has the appropriate software, the image quality may be improved and synchronisation errors amended through the ECG editing tools (ignore premature beats, pacemaker spikes, etc.). The definitive analysis is performed using the cardiac CT workstation's specialised software. First, the axial images must be examined, with different window adjustments (pulmonary, mediastinum window level, etc.) to perform an adequate assessment of the entire anatomical structure of the thoracic volume acquired. The coronary analysis must include oblique multiplanar reconstructions (see Chap. 10, Figs. 10.6–10.8), which are particularly useful if there is marked calcification of the coronary vessel wall, in which the maximum intensity projections (MIP) can be unclear unless they are performed with very thin slices. These MIP are more useful for evaluating the coronary lumen, and the possible presence of vessel stenosis, in the absence of calcification, and offer a suitable emulation of the invasive angiography when combined with three-dimensional reconstructions (see Chap. 10, Fig. 10.11). The 3D *volume-rendering* image is useful for visualising the distribution of the coronary arteries (see Chap. 10, Fig. 10.13), studying anomalies in the origin and course of the coronary arteries and for quick detection of areas with possible obstructive lesions, although not for evaluating their magnitude.

- *Report*: must include the clinical indication for the examination and the basic technical details (type of acquisition, slice thickness, contrast volume, etc.). The pattern of coronary dominance will be indicated, and the findings in the various vessels and segments will be reported, according to the 17-segment coronary artery scheme of the American Heart Association. The assessment of the stenosis can be made with a quantitative comparative analysis (QCA) software, but this requires always a careful review and the appropriate manual correction when the automatic detection of the lumen of the vessel is inadequate. The direct visual assessment of the stenosis, which has been validated and is an accepted method, has been shown to have good agreement with invasive angiography. Lesions must be evaluated in at least two longitudinal orthogonal sections of the vessel, but the assessment of the minimal luminal area is also recommended in transverse sections, in particular in cases of stenosis of borderline or indeterminate severity. According to the guidelines, the magnitude of the lesion should be classified as normal lesions (no atheromatous plaque, no stenosis), minimal lesions (plaque with <25 % stenosis), mild lesions (25–49 % stenosis), moderate lesions (50–60 % stenosis), significant or severe lesions (70–99 % stenosis) or vessel occlusion (100 % stenosis). It is also recommended to report the composition of the most significant lesions as calcified (see Fig. 9.3a), non-calcified (see Fig. 9.3b) or mixed plaque, the distribution of the lesion along the vessel wall (concentric, eccentric), its location in the course of the vessel (proximal, medial, distal, diffuse, ostial, bifurcational, intrastent, etc.) and the presence of vessel remodelling. Finally, the report must include a section where possible extracoronary findings are described (cardiac and extracardiac) as well as a final clinical orientation based on the findings of the study and the context of the patient.

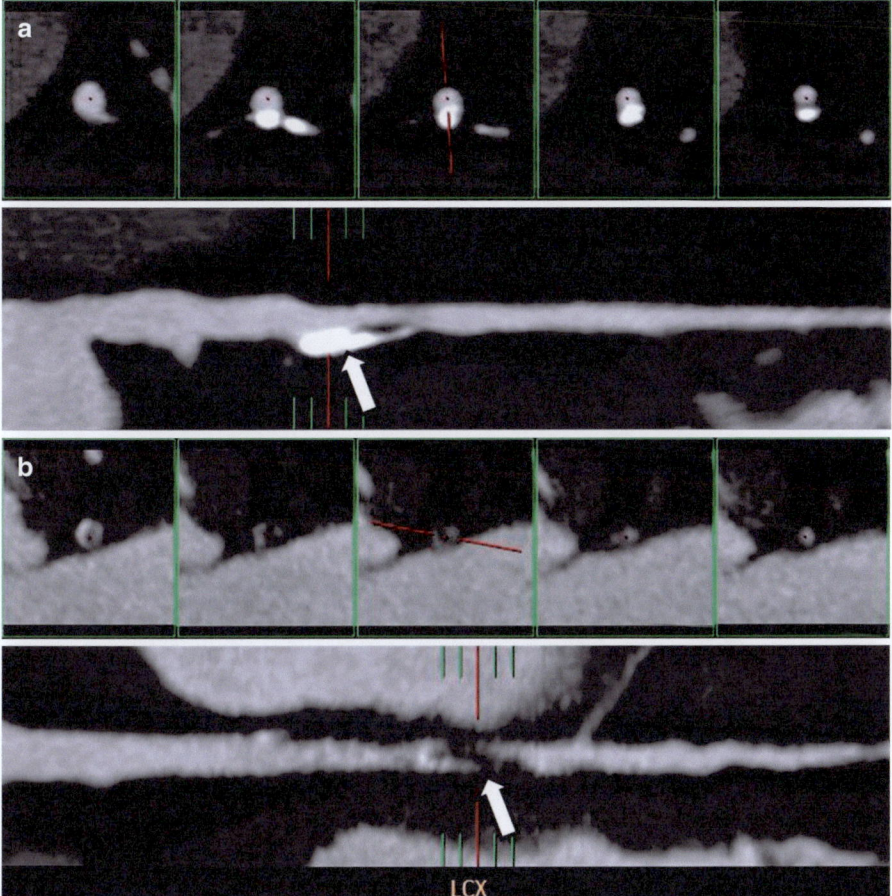

Fig. 9.3 Examples of calcified (**a**) and non-calcified (**b**) coronary artery lesions (*arrows*)

9.4.3 Triple Rule-Out MDCT Study

Triple rule-out studies by MDCT are examinations performed with electrocardiographic synchronisation that allow the pulmonary arteries and the lung parenchyma to be assessed (see Fig. 9.4a) along with the coronary vessels and the thoracic aorta (see Fig. 9.4b). They are used mainly in emergency departments in patients with chest pain in whom a distinction between three diagnostic options is required: acute coronary syndrome, acute aortic syndrome and pulmonary thromboembolism.

The preparation of the patient is similar to conventional coronary MDCT. If the patient is unable to perform an adequate breath hold, the study may be performed in the caudo-cranial direction in order to minimise movement artefacts due to respiration.

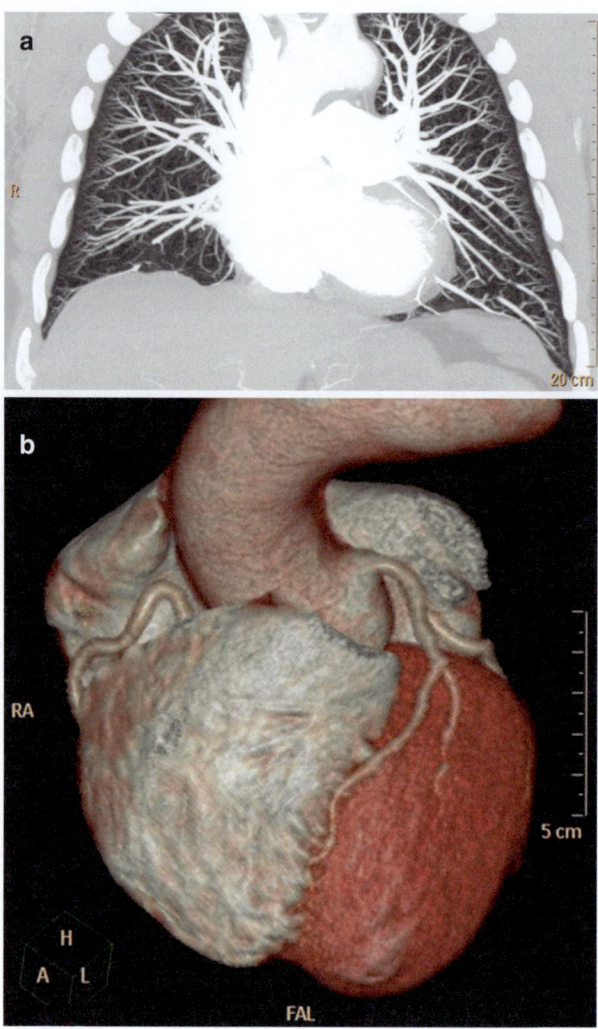

Fig. 9.4 CT acquisitions for a triple rule-out study including pulmonary arteries (**a**) and aorta and coronary vessels (**b**)

In triple rule-out studies, the acquisition must be performed from the lower border of the collarbones, approximately 20 mm above the upper border of the aortic arch down to the upper third of the abdomen. Contrast is injected in biphasic mode whenever possible. In the first phase, 70–80 ml of contrast is injected at a speed of 5 ml/s and, in the second, 50–60 ml of diluted contrast (25–30 ml contrast + 25–30 ml saline solution). If this is not possible, 100–120 ml of iodine contrast may be injected at a speed of 5 ml/s without additional saline solution to avoid the washout of the contrast from the right heart cavities. The field of view should include the whole thorax, not just the heart. The rest of the protocol is similar to that followed in conventional coronary MDCT.

9.4.4 Study of Pulmonary Veins

MDCT studies of the pulmonary veins are indicated in patients with atrial fibrillation on whom an ablation of the pulmonary vein ostia is going to be performed.

The examination will be carried out with electrocardiographic synchronisation. Although various protocols have been described, in order to simplify the studies, the protocol for the injection of contrast and of acquisition can be the same as that of non-invasive coronary catheterisation.

The identification of the number and the arrangement of the pulmonary veins and their ostia (see Fig. 9.5) and the possibility of integrating the image with the programmes of electrophysiological mapping of the atria are very useful for planning procedures in this type of patient.

9.4.5 Study of Cardiac Veins

Knowledge of the anatomy of the cardiac veins is very important in those patients in whom resynchronisation therapy is considered, which requires the insertion of electrodes of epicardial stimulation of the left ventricle by way of a cardiac vein (see Fig. 9.6). The acquisition protocol of the images is again the same as that of MDCT studies of the coronary arteries, and only the protocol for the injection of contrast needs to be changed. In these cases, the injection of at least 100 ml of contrast at a speed of 4 ml/s is recommended or a biphasic injection of 30 ml at 3 ml/s followed by 70 ml at 5 ml/s and then 40 ml of saline solution at 5 ml/s for flushing.

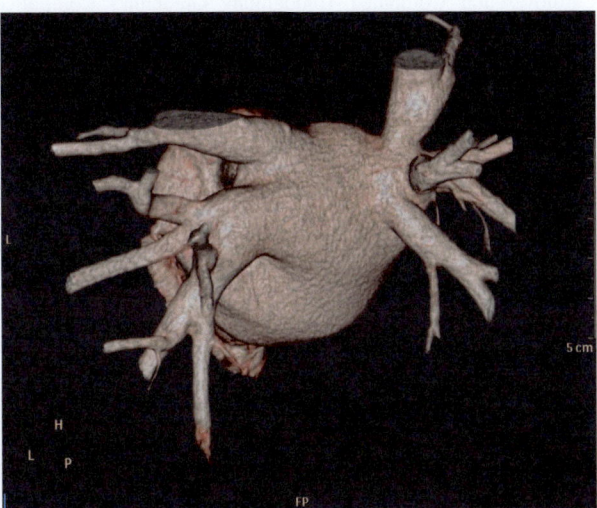

Fig. 9.5 3D reconstruction of a CT study of pulmonary veins

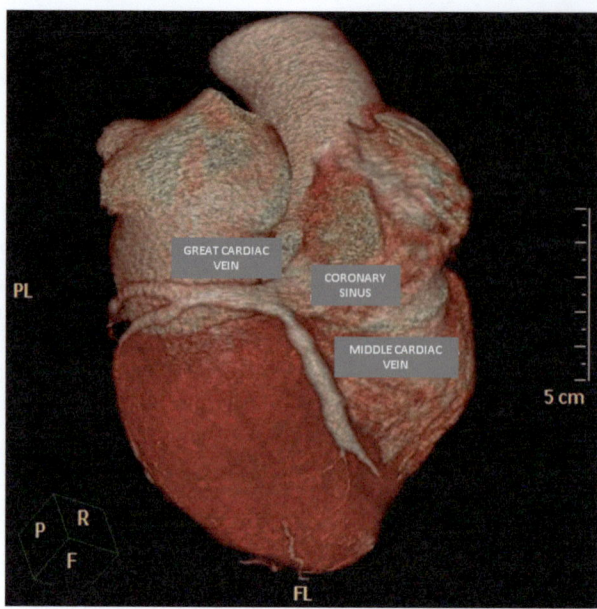

Fig. 9.6 Posterior view of the heart from a 3D reconstruction where the coronary veins are visualised

Recommended Bibliography

1. Abbara S, Arbab-Zadeh A, Callister TQ, Desai MY, Mamuya W, Thomson L et al (2009) SCCT guidelines for performance of coronary computed tomographic angiography: a report of the Society of Cardiovascular Computed Tomography Guidelines Committee. J Cardiovasc Comput Tomogr 3:190–204
2. Kramer CM, Budoff MJ, Fayad ZA, Ferrari VA, Goldman C, Lesser JR et al (2007) ACCF/AHA 2007 clinical competence statement on vascular imaging with computed tomography and magnetic resonance. A report of the American College of Cardiology Foundation/American Heart Association/American College of Physicians Task Force on Clinical Competence and Training. J Am Coll Cardiol 50:1097–1114
3. Lin EC (2007) Coronary computed tomography angiography: principles of contrast material administration. J Cardiovasc Comput Tomogr 1:162–165
4. Maroules CD, Cheezum MK, Joshi PH, Williams M, Simprini LA, Nelson KH et al (2015) SCCT curriculum guidelines for general (level 1) cardiovascular CT training. J Cardiovasc Comput Tomogr 9:81–88
5. Taylor AJ, Cerqueira M, Hodgson JM, Mark D, Min J, O'Gara P et al (2010) ACCF/SCCT/ACR/AHA/ASE/ASNC/NASCI/SCAI/SCMR 2010 appropriate use criteria for cardiac computed tomography. J Am Coll Cardiol 56:1864–1894

Cardiac Computed Tomography: Post-processing and Analysis

10

Rubén Leta and Antonio Barros

10.1 Introduction

Careful acquisition of studies is essential for obtaining images of the cardiac anatomy that are adequate for analysis.

The process of analysis begins at the main console of the system with a first, quick visualisation of the axial images aimed to ensure, while the patient is still in the examination room, that the study is adequate and there is no need for repeat acquisition. In this sense, it is worth evaluating the correct contrast of the cardiac structures, as well as the presence of respiratory motion artefacts (see Fig. 10.1, arrows), which are problems that cannot be solved by post-processing tools. Also, early detection of cardiac motion artefacts due to a defective synchronisation (see Fig. 10.2a) may prompt additional reconstructions to be performed at the console with the help of software for editing of the ECG signal reference (see Fig. 10.2b).

This first analysis of axial images is also useful for excluding extracardiac findings, some of which may be important enough to extend the acquisition, such as, for example, the unexpected finding of thoracic aorta dissection, for which additional abdominal and iliac sections should be taken. In this sense, a systematic stepwise analysis of the cardiac and thoracic anatomy is essential in order not to overlook important findings: lung parenchyma, respiratory tract, large pulmonary vessels, large systemic vessels and so on.

R. Leta, MD, PhD (✉) • Antonio Barros, MD
Cardiac Imaging Unit, Cardiology Department, Hospital de la Santa Creu i Sant Pau, Universitat Autònoma de Barcelona, Barcelona, Spain
e-mail: rleta@santpau.cat

© Springer International Publishing Switzerland 2016
G. Pons-Lladó (ed.), *Protocols for Cardiac MR and CT*,
DOI 10.1007/978-3-319-30831-9_10

Fig. 10.1 Detection of artefacts due to respiratory motion (*arrows*) in a cardiac CT study

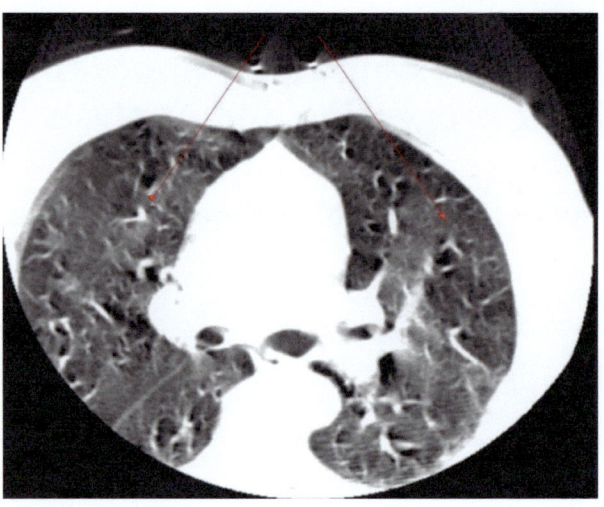

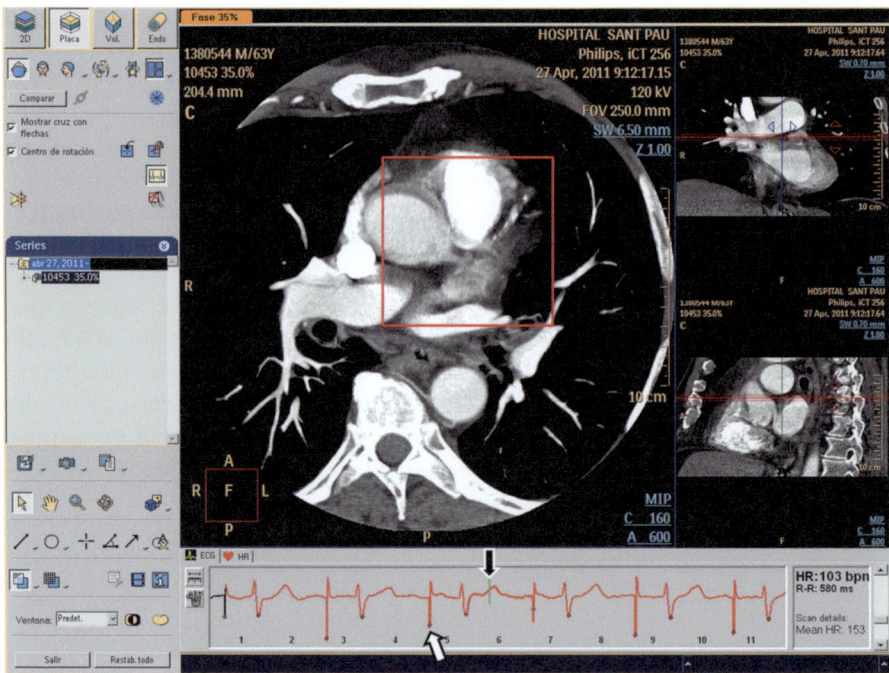

Fig. 10.2 (**a**). Reconstruction artefact (*squared box*) after a synchronisation with the atrial stimulation signal of a pacemaker (*white arrow on the ECG line*) leading to an inappropriate cardiac phase (*black arrow*). (**b**). Manual editing of the reference ECG with selection of a true QRS complex (*white arrow on the ECG line*) that allows for an appropriate cardiac phase to be chosen (*black arrow*), with subsequent correction of the artefact (*squared box*)

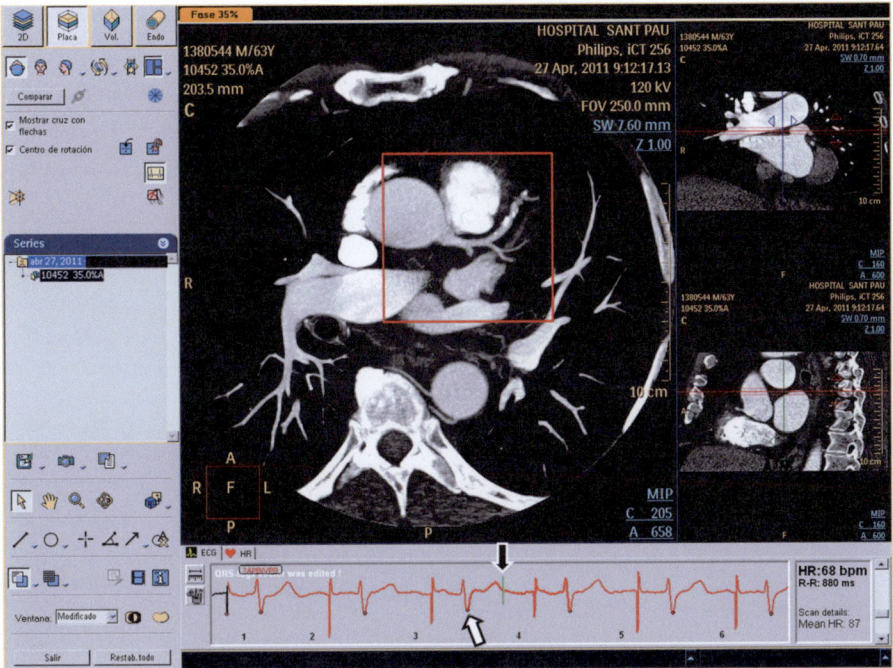

Fig. 10.2 (continued)

10.2 Analysis Tools

After the pre-visualisation in the acquisition console, the analysis of the cardiac CT study is completed at the post-processing workstations. Though the various commercial analysis systems may differ, they share some common visualisation tools which provide several modes of image reconstruction. The examination of the native axial images themselves, however, remains essential for starting the analysis.

10.2.1 Axial Images

As the acquisition in CT systems is made on axial planes, images in this orientation do not suffer from the reconstruction artefacts that, in greater or lesser degree, may affect multiplanar reconstruction images. The evaluation of possible interference due to heart movement on the axial images, particularly in cardiac studies with helical acquisition, is important for choosing the most adequate phase of the cardiac cycle to be analysed.

To speed up the analysis, it is common for post-processing stations to perform a "segmentation" of the anatomy (see Fig. 10.3), which consists of enhancing certain

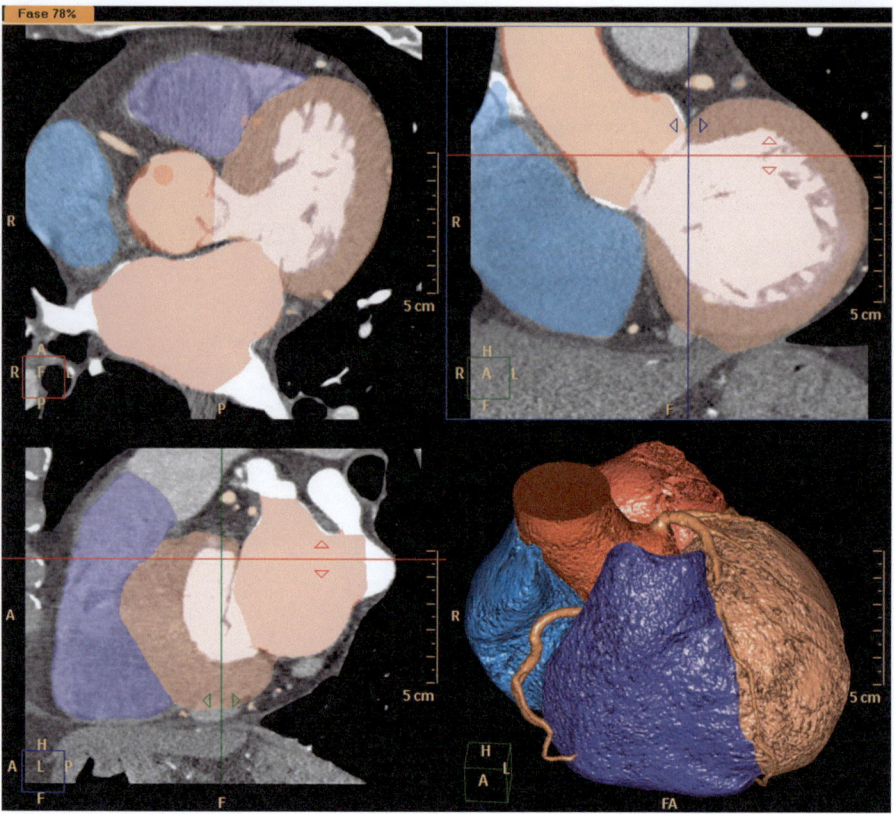

Fig. 10.3 Computerised post-processing analysis with segmentation of cardiac structures

anatomical structures in the images, while attenuating others of lesser interest for cardiac studies. This computer process has potential limitations as it may lead to an unwanted loss of visualisation of structures that could be important to analyse. This is an additional reason for relying on the visualisation of the axial images, which contain all the information acquired and not only that presented by the workstation after post-processing.

10.2.2 Multiplane Images

As the acquisition of CT systems is on an axial orientation, any image that is not shown on the axial plane must correspond to a reconstruction from multiple axial planes. These are known as multiplanar reconstruction (MPR) images, which include oblique and, also, strict sagittal and coronal planes. Two types of MPR reconstruction are available: oblique and curved.

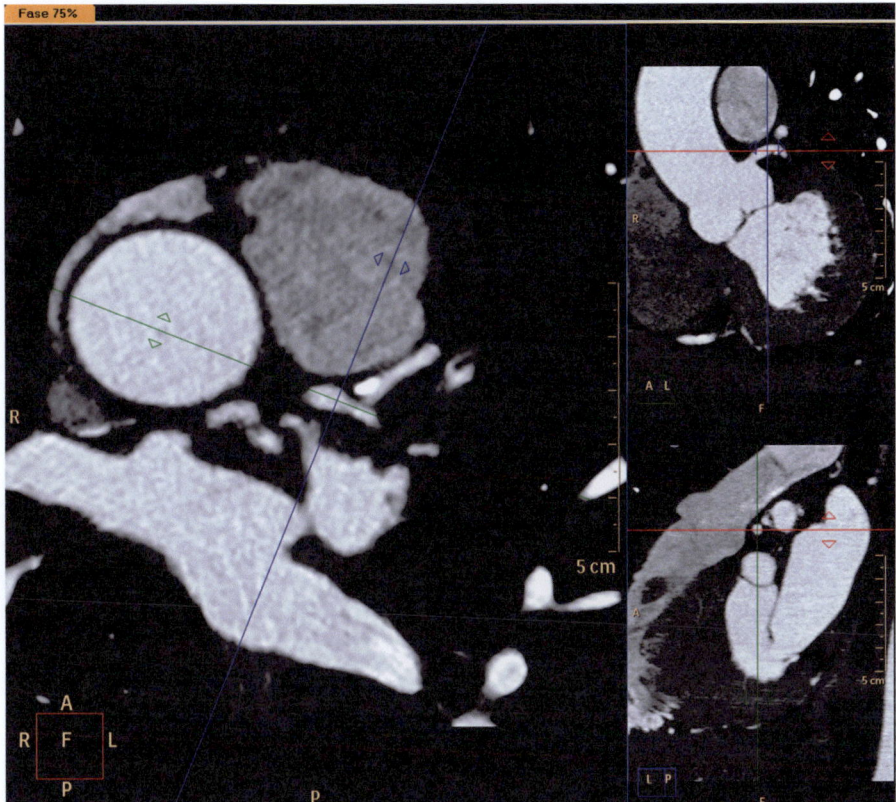

Fig. 10.4 Tools for manual obtention of oblique MPR slices oriented on anatomical planes of individual coronary arteries

10.2.2.1 Oblique MPR

In this mode (see Fig. 10.4), images are acquired using computer reconstruction through the angulation of two planes perpendicular to the axial plane, keeping an angle of 90° between them, such as images in coronal and sagittal sections, as well as the various intermediate angulations between them. This type of reconstruction is useful for obtaining transverse sections of the coronary arteries (see Fig. 10.5), from which important information may be drawn, such as the minimal luminal area, which determines the significance of a lesion or the presence of vascular remodelling. These planes, which are cross-sectional to the vessel, are known as "*IVUS-like*" given their similarity to the images obtained by intravascular ultrasound, although with lower resolution.

10.2.2.2 Curved MPRs

This mode of reconstruction (see Fig. 10.6) provides a longitudinal view of any vascular structure (coronary arteries, aorta, etc.). The image results from the spatial summation of those voxels of the axial plane that contain information on the

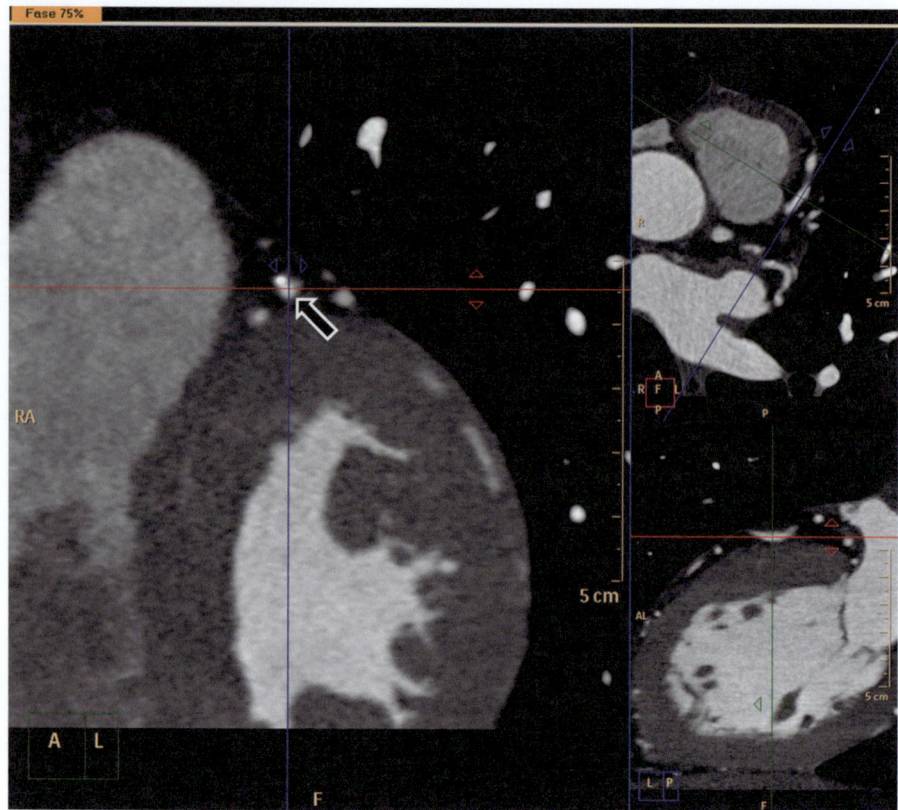

Fig. 10.5 Cross-sectional view of the left anterior descending coronary artery (*arrow*) obtained by oblique MPR analysis

anatomical structure of interest. These voxels are linked by the so-called centre line (see Fig. 10.7), which is drawn by the operator either by hand or semi-automatically. The vascular structure represented through curved MPR may be additionally post-processed to obtain transverse sections of the vessel (e.g. IVUS-like) or to visualise longitudinal sections with different angulations (see Fig. 10.8). These reconstructions are very useful for examining the coronary lumen and quantifying the magnitude of stenoses, in particular if there is vessel wall calcification. As with oblique MPR reconstructions, the curved representations are very useful tools for analysing the morphology and composition of coronary atheroma plaque.

Both the axial images and the multiplanar reconstructions are, in fact, two-dimensional sections. Nevertheless, post-processing tools also allow three-dimensional (3D) reconstructions of the cardiac structures to be obtained by computation of processes of spatial summation of consecutive axial slices. The resultant volume is useful for visual analysis, but the additional application of other post-processing tools on it is required to complete the analysis.

Fig. 10.6 Curved MPR of the left anterior descending coronary artery

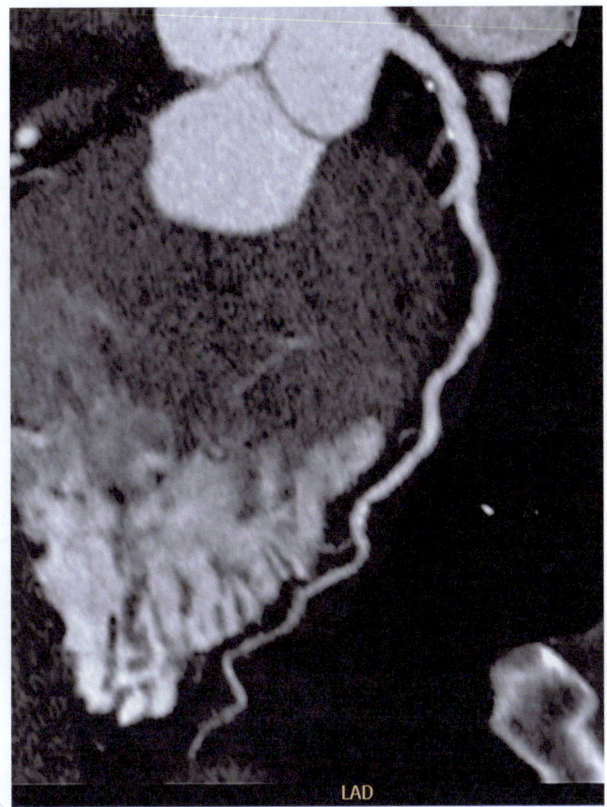

10.2.3 Other Post-processing Tools

Other post-processing tools that have shown their usefulness in cardiac CT analysis are maximum intensity projection (MIP), minimum intensity projection (MinIP) and volume render images. These tools can be applied on axial images, multiplanar slices or 3D reconstructions.

10.2.3.1 MIP and MinIP

In MIP images (see Fig. 10.9), again a spatial summation of slices is performed, in this case highlighting those structures with the highest density or, in other words, with the highest ray attenuation power (e.g. vessels with contrast), which are "projected" in close up, whatever their actual spatial situation. Conversely, in the MinIP images (see Fig. 10.10), the reconstruction gives more prominence to structures with lower density, or attenuation (e.g. the respiratory system), which are highlighted in relation to the rest of tissues.

MIP mode, when applied to MPR or 3D reconstructions, offers a fairly good simulation of an invasive coronary angiography (see Fig. 10.11), which is itself also a spatial projection image. MIP images are also useful in the detection of pulmonary

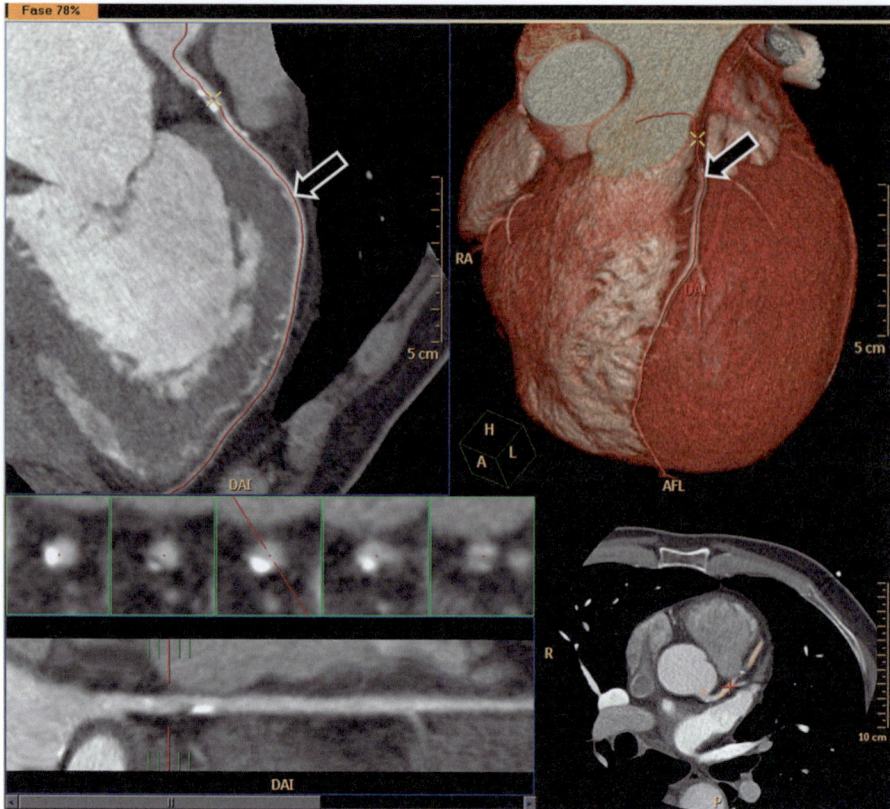

Fig. 10.7 Curved MPR of a left anterior descending coronary artery obtained by drawing of a line centred on the vessel lumen (*arrows*)

nodules, which may occasionally pass unnoticed in thin slices without MIP. Likewise, MinIP images are useful for visualising myocardial perfusion defects (see Fig. 10.12, arrows) and for detecting areas of pulmonary emphysema.

10.2.3.2 Volume Render

"Rendering" is a complex calculation process performed by a computer to generate a 2D image from a 3D model. In this mode of post-processing, the pixel intensity of the 2D images corresponds to the 3D voxel attenuation value represented (higher density shows up as brighter signal), but to which a correction factor is applied depending on the relative position of this voxel within the volume represented: given two structures with equivalent attenuation power, that located at a more superficial plane will be represented with brighter pixels. A 3D reconstruction with this type of post-processing is known as a 3D volume rendering image (Fig. 10.13). This mode of reconstruction allows a quick visualisation of the coronary anatomy and the distribution of the vessels on the epicardial surface of the heart, which may allow the localisation at first sight of obstructive coronary lesions and congenital

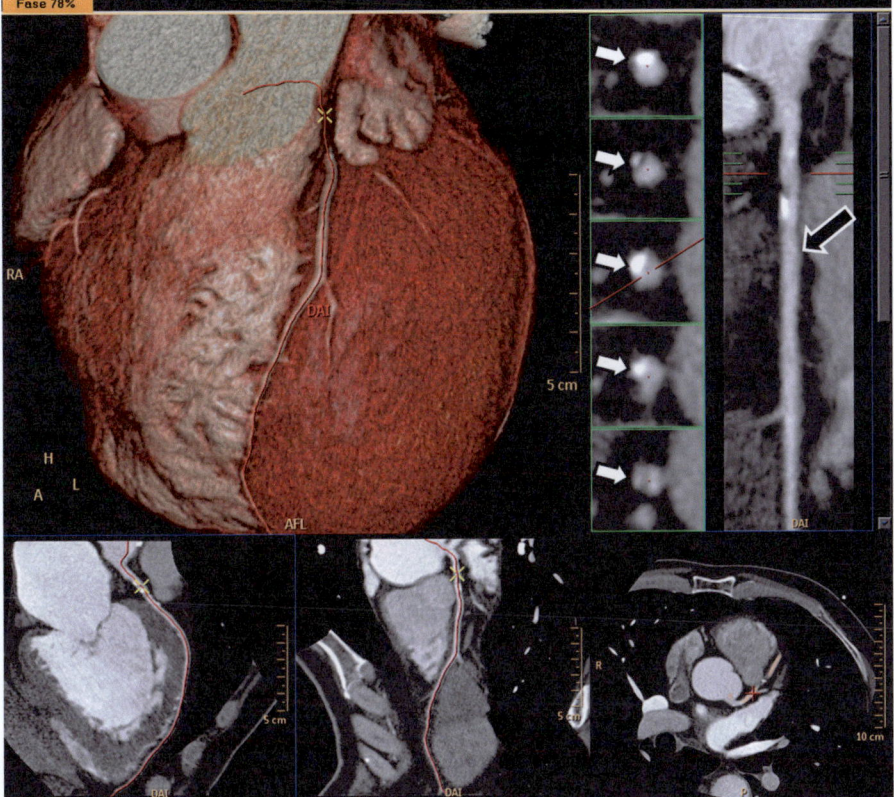

Fig. 10.8 Transverse (*white arrows*) and longitudinal (*black arrow*) views of a left anterior descending coronary artery obtained by curved MPR

anomalies of the vessels. Despite their appeal, 3D-rendered images are not the most suitable for assessing the magnitude of coronary stenoses, in particular when there are calcium components in the lesion (see Fig. 10.14, arrow on the left panel), which, in this type of post-processing, can mask the actual significance of the obstruction, and lead to discrepancies with invasive angiography (see Fig. 10.14, arrow in the right panel).

10.3 Evaluation of the Magnitude and Composition of Coronary Lesions

The study of the anatomy of the coronary arteries by MDCT has great potential for information that is not limited to the lumen of the vessels but also to their walls. Thus, the examination can evaluate both the stenosis caused by coronary lesions and the distribution, composition and morphology of the plaques themselves.

Fig. 10.9 MIP image of axial slices from a cardiac CT study

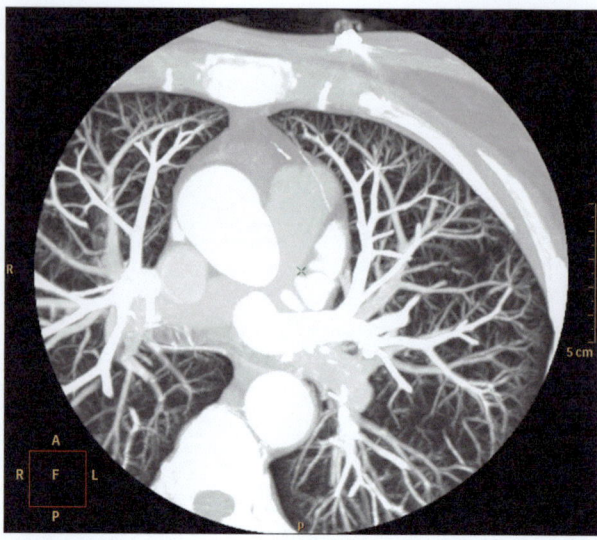

Fig. 10.10 MinIP image of axial slices from a cardiac CT study

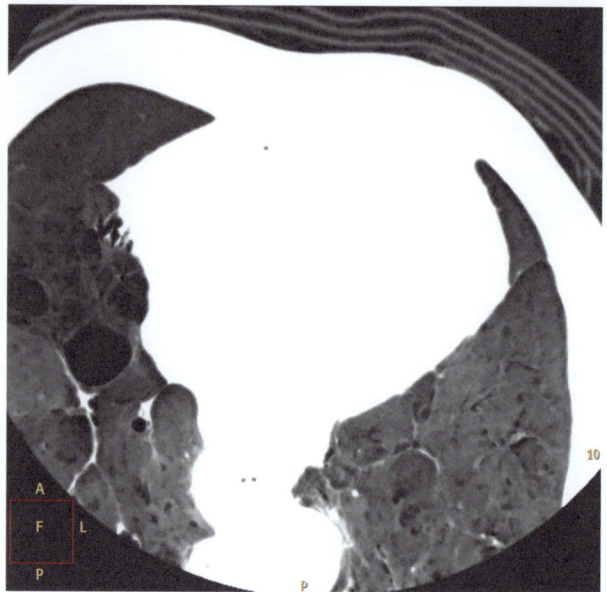

10.3.1 Evaluation of the Magnitude of the Lesions

A first aspect to consider once a lesion is detected is to ensure that the finding truly corresponds to a lesion and not to an artefact. The most frequent causes of artefacts are cardiac and respiratory movements, which may cause pseudostenosis (see Fig. 10.15, arrow in the left panel); the analysis tools themselves, causing

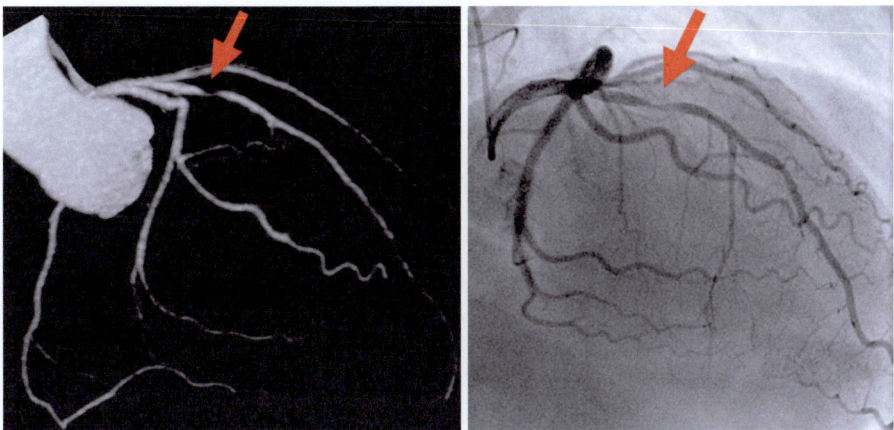

Fig. 10.11 3D MIP reconstruction (*left panel*) showing a stenotic lesion at the left anterior descending (*arrow*) and the correspondent invasive angiography image (*right panel*) for comparison

Fig. 10.12 MIP reconstruction of the left ventricle in coronal plane showing extensive myocardial perfusion defects (*arrows*) in a patient with ischemic heart disease

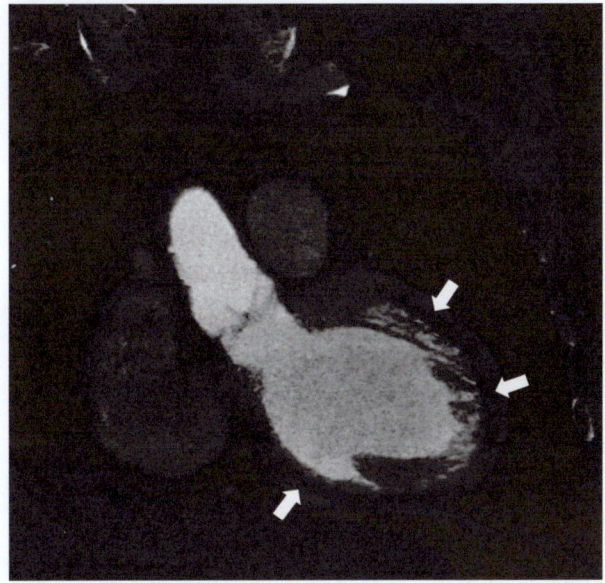

pseudostenosis due to incorrect positioning of the centre line (see Fig. 10.16); and the partial volume effect due to significant coronary wall calcification (See Fig. 10.17).

The evaluation of coronary stenosis by cardiac MDCT (just as with invasive coronary catheterisation) is performed taking into account the magnitude of the reduction of the diameter of the vessel lumen in the lesion (minimal luminal diameter) relative to an adjacent segment free of lesions, which is taken as a

Fig. 10.13 Frontal view of a 3D volume rendering of the heart

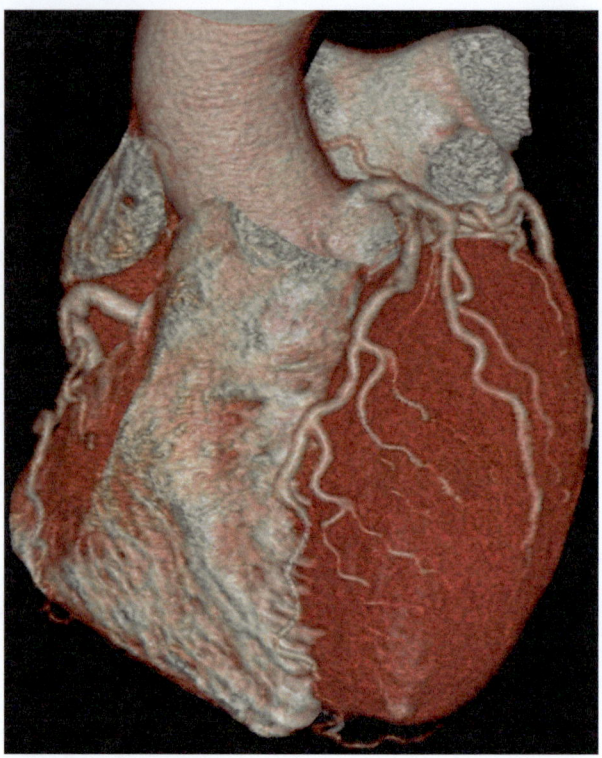

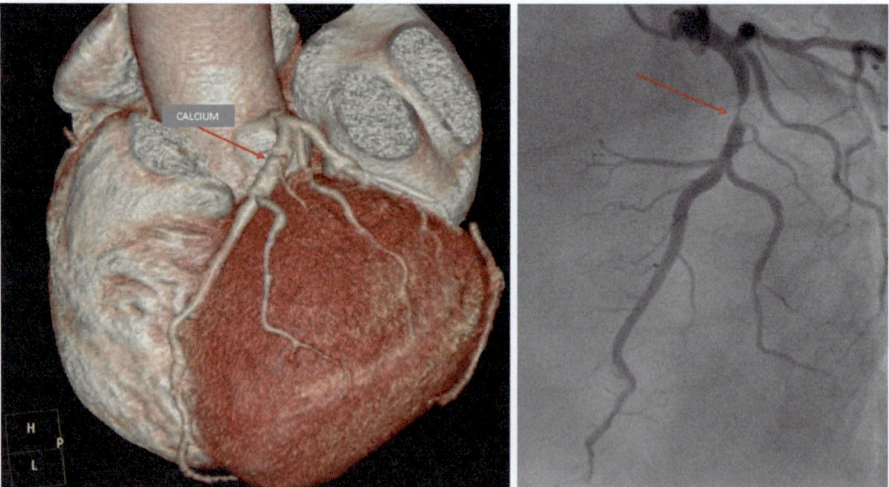

Fig. 10.14 3D volume rendering (*left panel*) showing calcification of the left anterior descending artery precluding the detection of an underlying severely obstructed lesion, as shown in the invasive angiography (*arrow*, in the *right panel*)

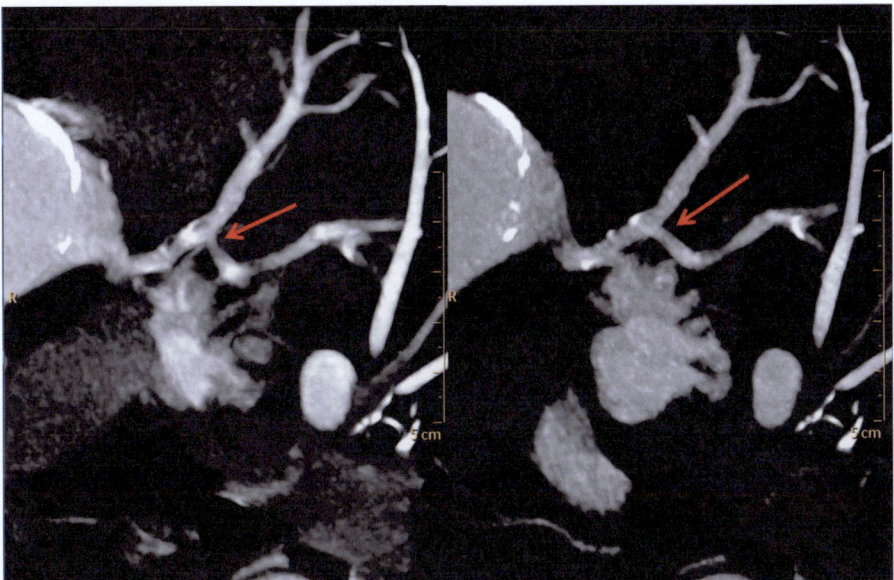

Fig. 10.15 False stenosis (*arrow, left panel*) due to cardiac motion artefact on an otherwise normal vessel, as proven with the analysis of a more appropriate cardiac phase (*right panel*)

reference. Just as in the invasive study, this evaluation can be performed visually, although current cardiac MDCT analysis stations use specialised software to quantify the degree of obstruction. On the one hand, these systems allow a totally automatic quantification, in which the borders of the arterial wall are detected (and, thus, the lumen of the vessel is delineated) (see Fig. 10.18a, b), and on the other hand, a semi-automatic quantification is also available, in which the user manually sets calibrating markers in both the lumen at the level of the lesion (see Fig. 10.19, lower arrow) and the reference segment of the vessel (see Fig. 10.19, upper arrow). The system then performs the calculation of the stenosis. It is important to bear in mind that with any automatic quantification system, a fundamental requirement is to have optimal image quality so that the detection of the borders of the wall and the quantification of the stenosis are reliable.

Also, multiplanar transverse reconstructions of the coronary arteries (IVUS-like) allow the quantification of the magnitude of the lesions by determining the minimal luminal area of the vessel at the site of maximal stenosis (see Fig. 10.18b), while the features of the coronary plaque may be also evaluated (see Fig. 10.20). This type of measurement not only requires optimal image quality but also an appropriate adjustment of the window parameters (level and thickness). Although this quantification can be applied to any lesions, the most difficult to analyse are those of intermediate significance, those located at the origin of the vessel (ostial) or cases when lesions

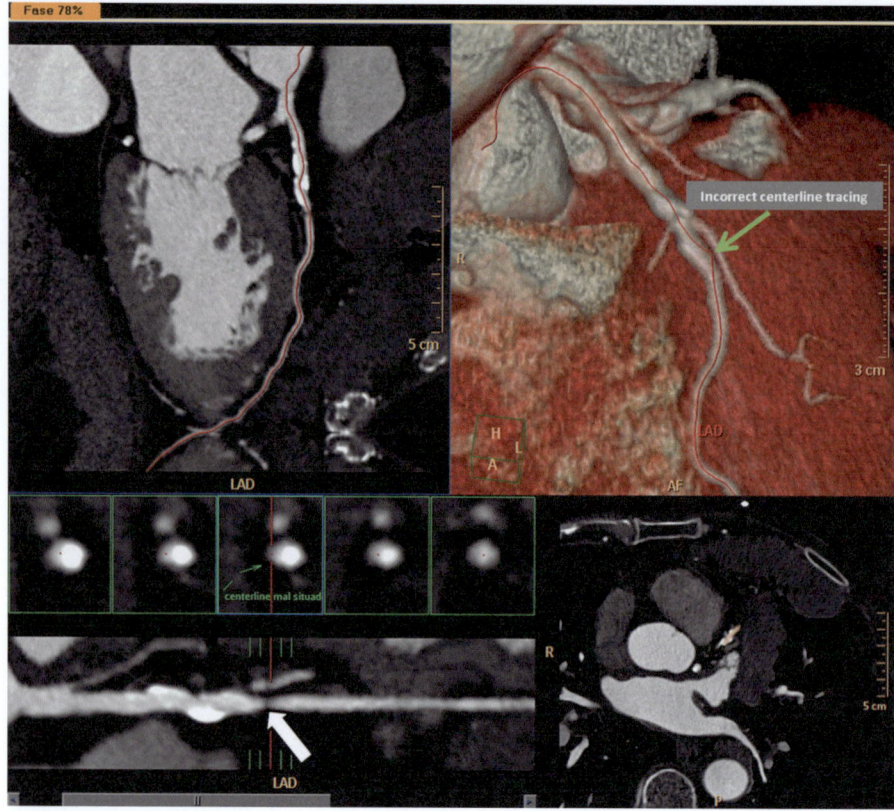

Fig. 10.16 False stenotic lesion on the MPR image (*white arrow*, in the *left lower panel*) due to an incorrect centre line tracing (*green arrow, in the right upper panel*)

are diffusely distributed, with no healthy segments to take as a reference (see Fig. 10.21a, b).

Current recommendations advocate quantifying the stenosis on a scale with relatively wide margins in the stenosis percentage, independently of the approach used for its evaluation (visual, automatic or semi-automatic).

10.3.2 Assessing Lesion Composition

Cardiac MDCT provides information on the components of the atherosclerotic plaque of which coronary lesions are constituted, based on their value in Hounsfield units (HU). This value expresses the magnitude with which the tissues are able to attenuate the X-rays emitted by an external source. By convention, a value of 0 has been established as that of the attenuation of water and, thus, more dense tissues, such as fibrous tissue or calcium, with progressively greater attenuation power, have higher HU values.

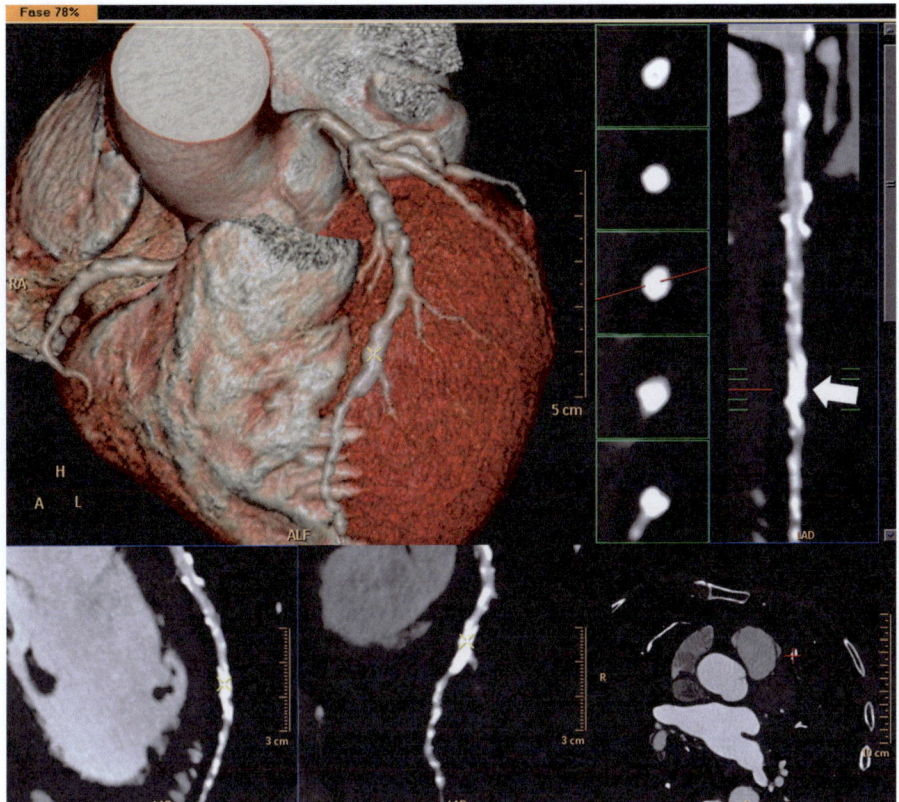

Fig. 10.17 Partial volume effect and blooming of the vessel lumen (*arrow*, in the *right upper panel*) due to extensive vessel wall calcification

Although it is possible to establish the predominant components of the plaque, scientific evidence of the clinical relevance of this information is still lacking. However, it is interesting to know that certain features detectable by MDCT have been described in the so-called vulnerable plaques: the type of vascular remodelling, the HU value of the plaque and the presence of spotty calcification in the centre of the atheroma plaque.

The phenomenon of vessel wall remodelling can be assessed by quantifying the vascular area in the region of the lesion in a transverse MPR section of the vessel, comparing it with the vascular area of an adjacent vessel segment without lesions (see Fig. 10.22). In vulnerable lesions, a phenomenon of positive remodelling has been observed, described by a ratio between both areas >1. Also, it has been documented that a potentially vulnerable atheroma is composed by a plaque showing <30 HU. The quantification of HU values can be made manually but requires the use of a region of interest of at least 0.1 mm^2 (see Fig. 10.23, arrows), carefully avoiding the inclusion in the measurement of the vessel lumen and the pericoronary fat tissue. Of particular interest is the detection of an area of very low density in the

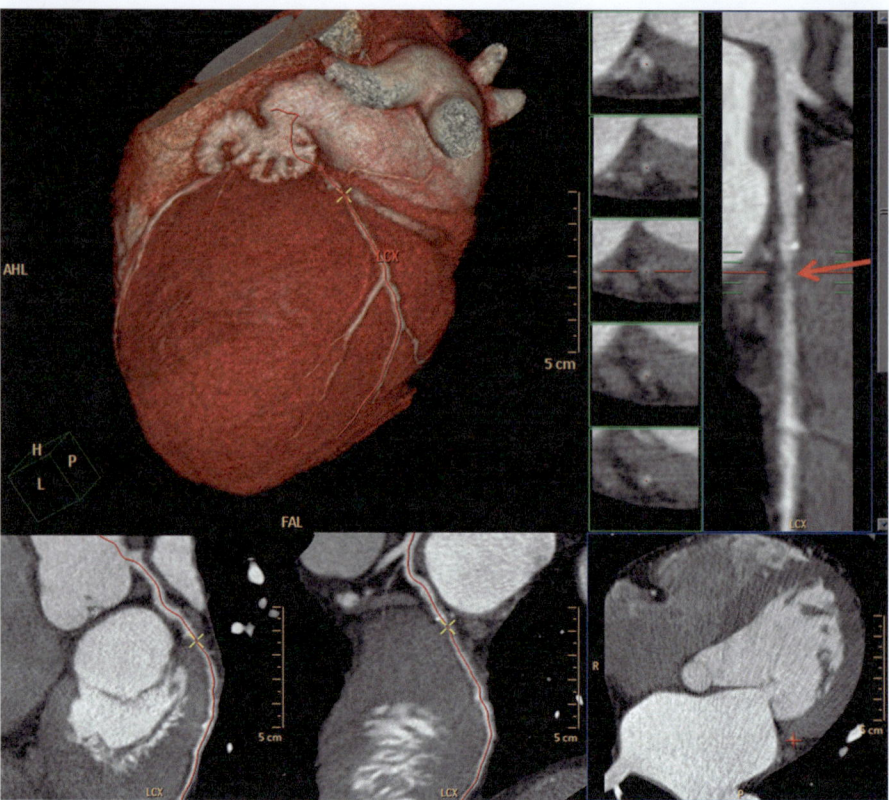

Fig. 10.18 (a) MPR showing an obstructive lesion of the circumflex artery (*arrow*). (b) Quantification of the degree of stenosis by automatic detection of the vessel borders, with calculation of the percentage of stenosis in terms of reduction of the diameter or the area of the vessel

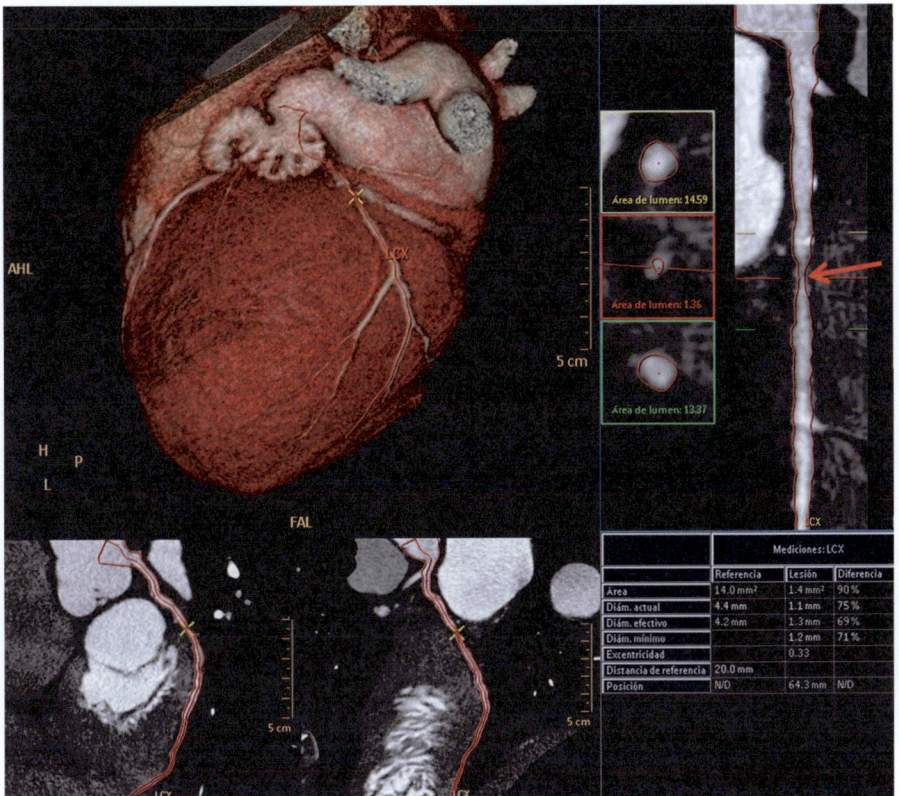

Fig. 10.18 (continued)

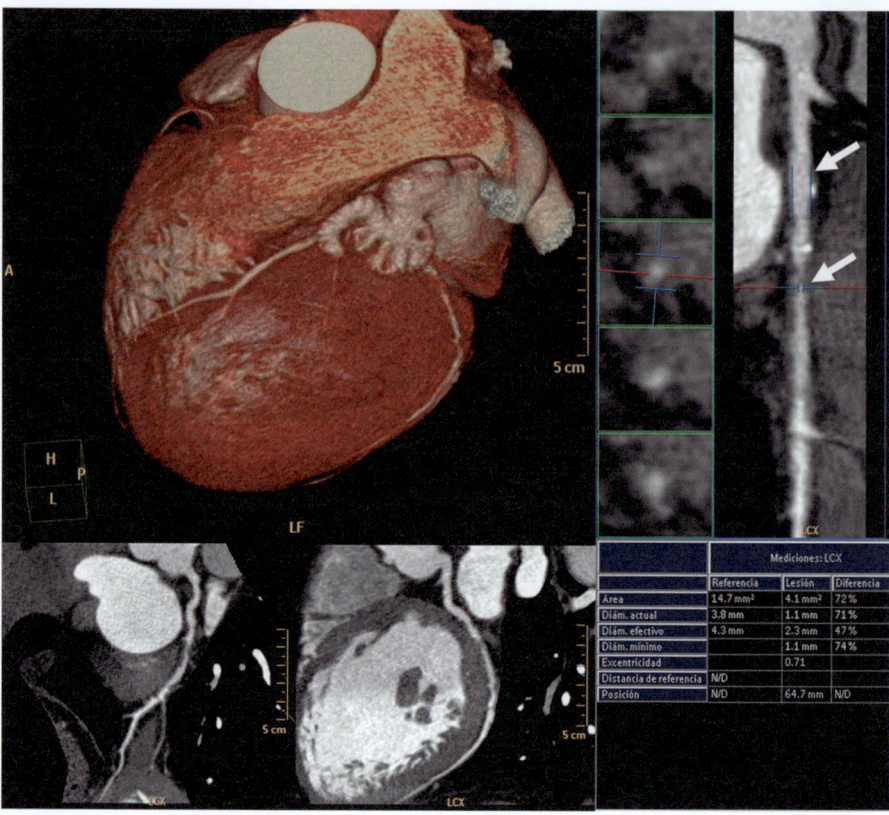

Fig. 10.19 Semi-automatic quantification of a lesion by manual setting of callipers at the site of obstruction (*lower arrow*, in the *right upper panel*), and at a healthy segment of the vessel (*upper arrow*), used as a reference

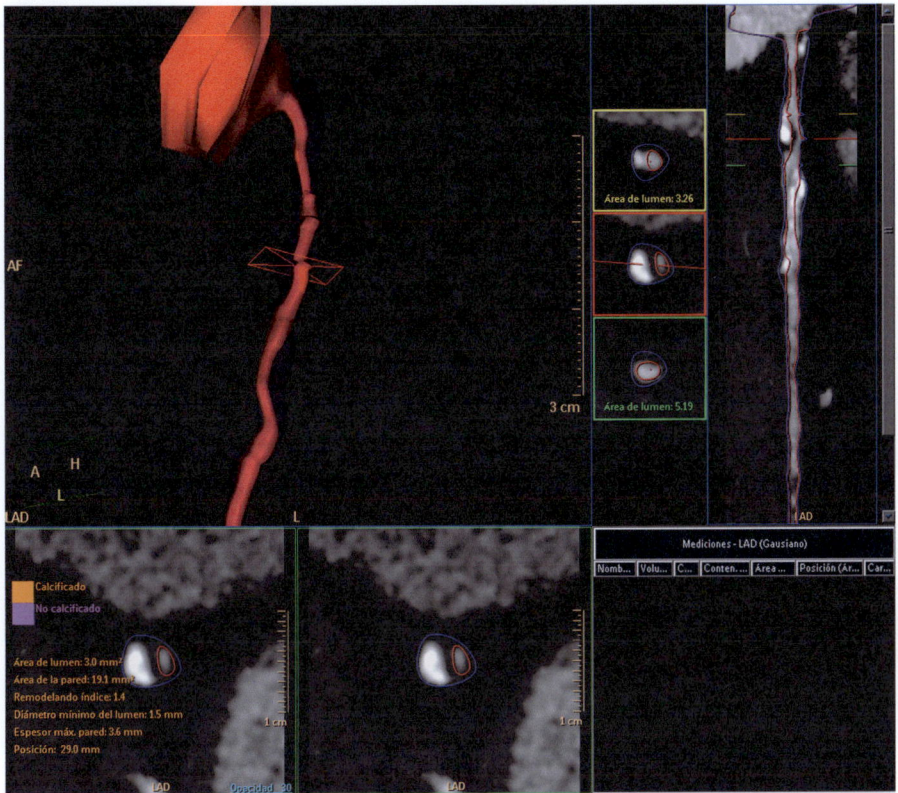

Fig. 10.20 High-quality cross-sectional images of a vessel at the site of a lesion (*lower panels*) where a morphological analysis of the components of the lesion can be performed, as well as quantitative measurements of vessel and lumen area

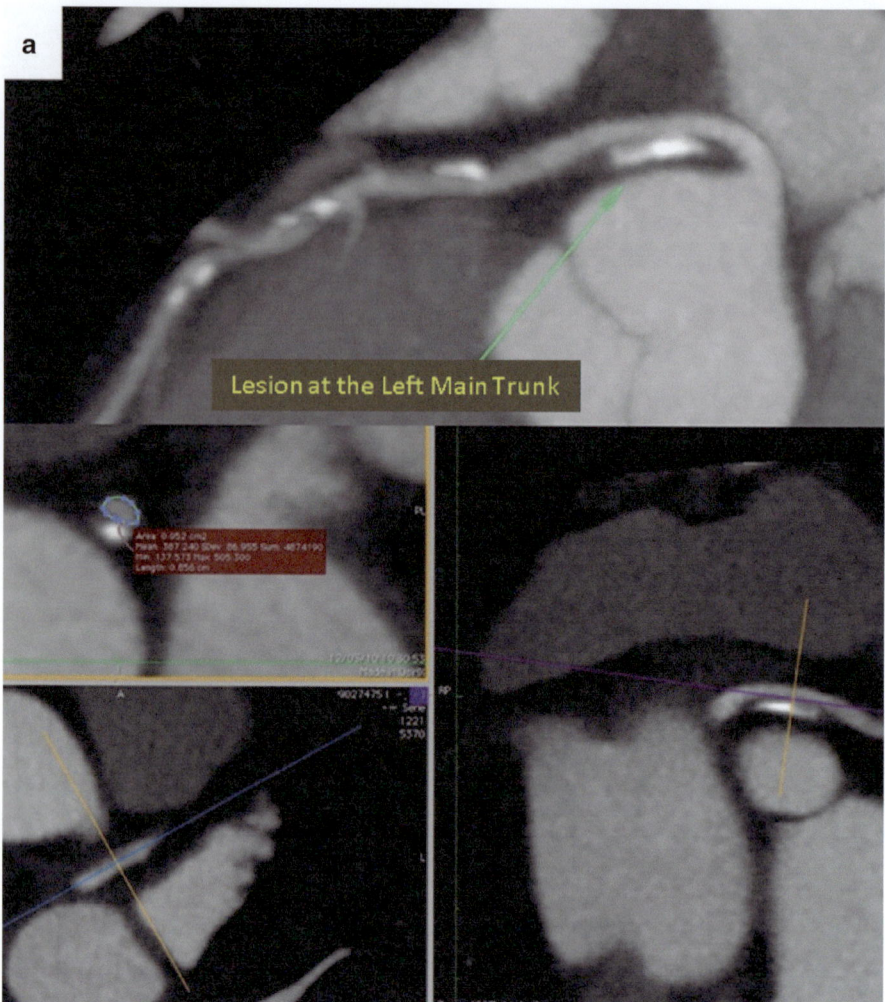

Fig. 10.21 Two examples (**a**, **b**) of diffuse lesions at the left main coronary artery (*green arrow, top panel in case* **a**) with limitations in their quantitative assessment due to the lack of a healthy vessel portion for reference. In these cases, absolute minimal area of the lumen vessel remains as the only element to assess the degree of obstruction: see the image from invasive angiography in case **b** (*red arrows, in lower right panel*)

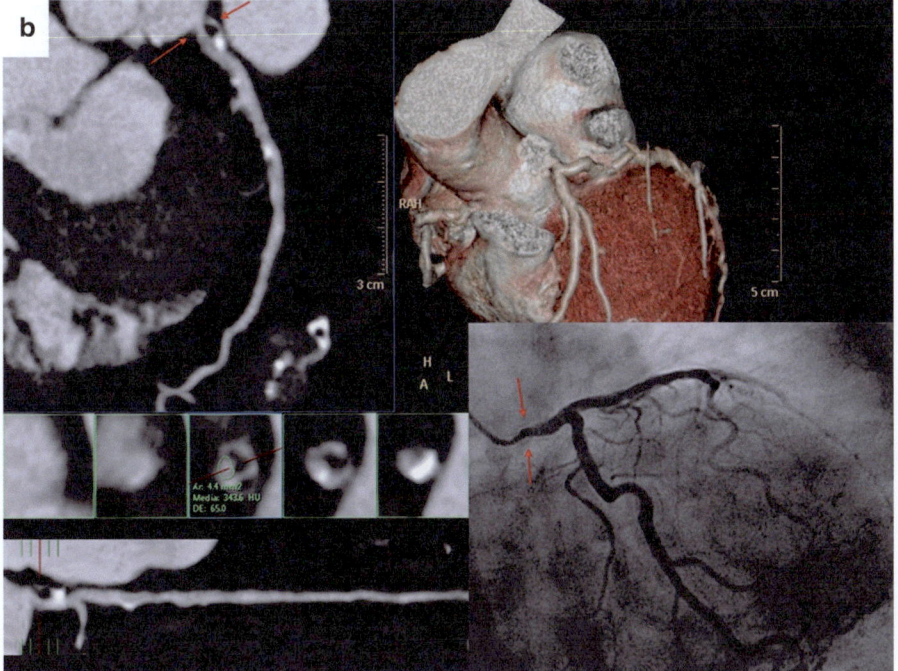

Fig. 10.21 (continued)

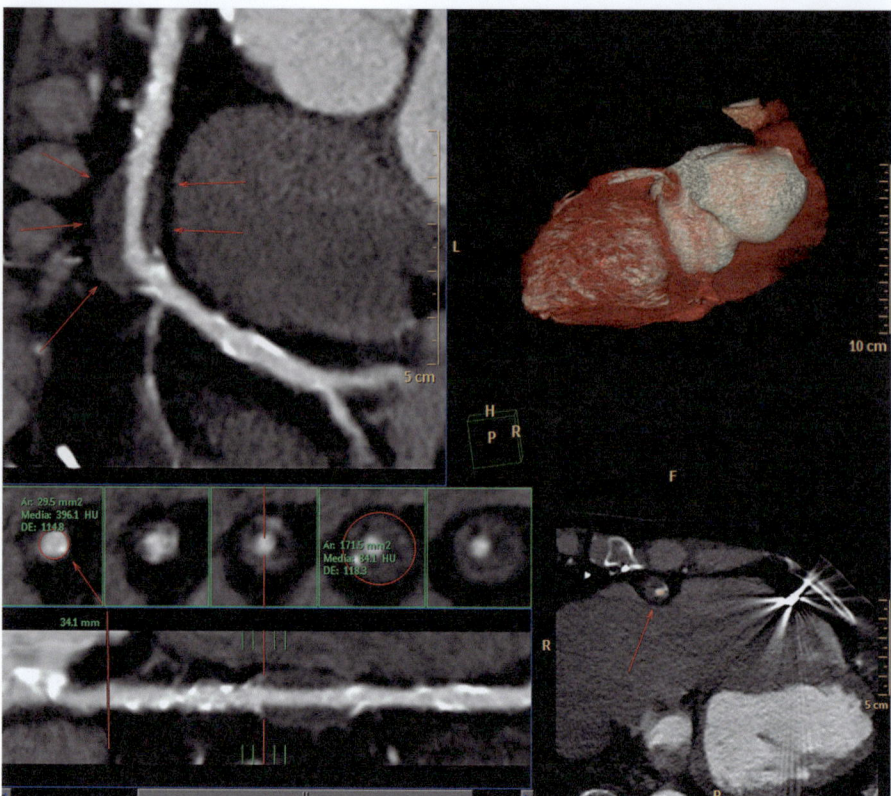

Fig. 10.22 Assessment of vascular remodelling by tracing of cross-sectional areas of the whole vessel at the involved site (*arrows*, in the *upper left panel*) and at a reference healthy segment: see circular areas at the middle left panel

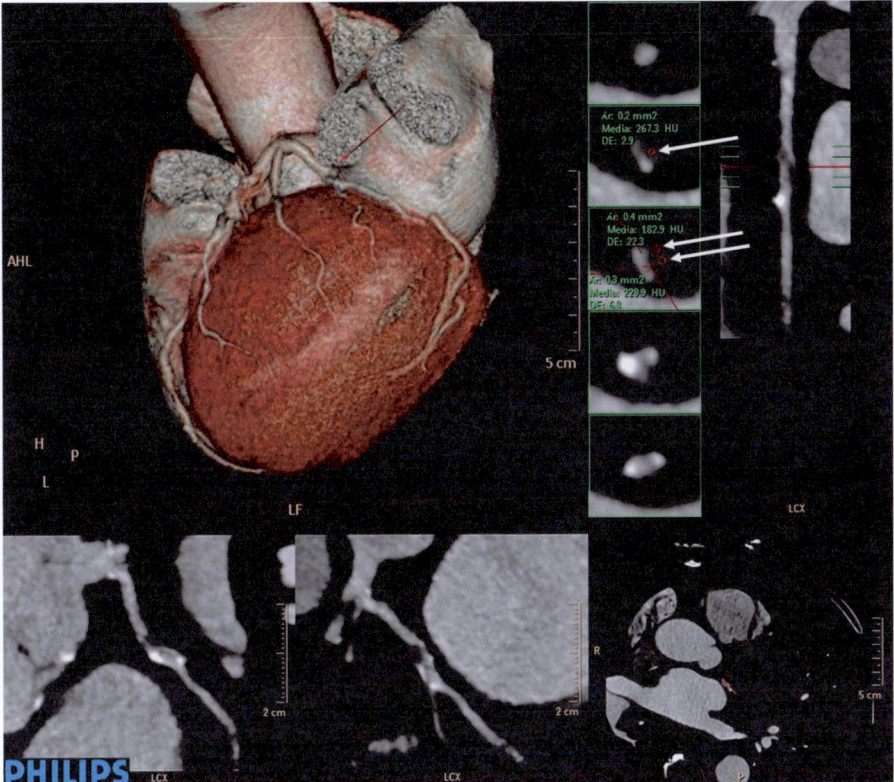

Fig. 10.23 Measurement of HU of the components of a coronary lesion (*arrows*)

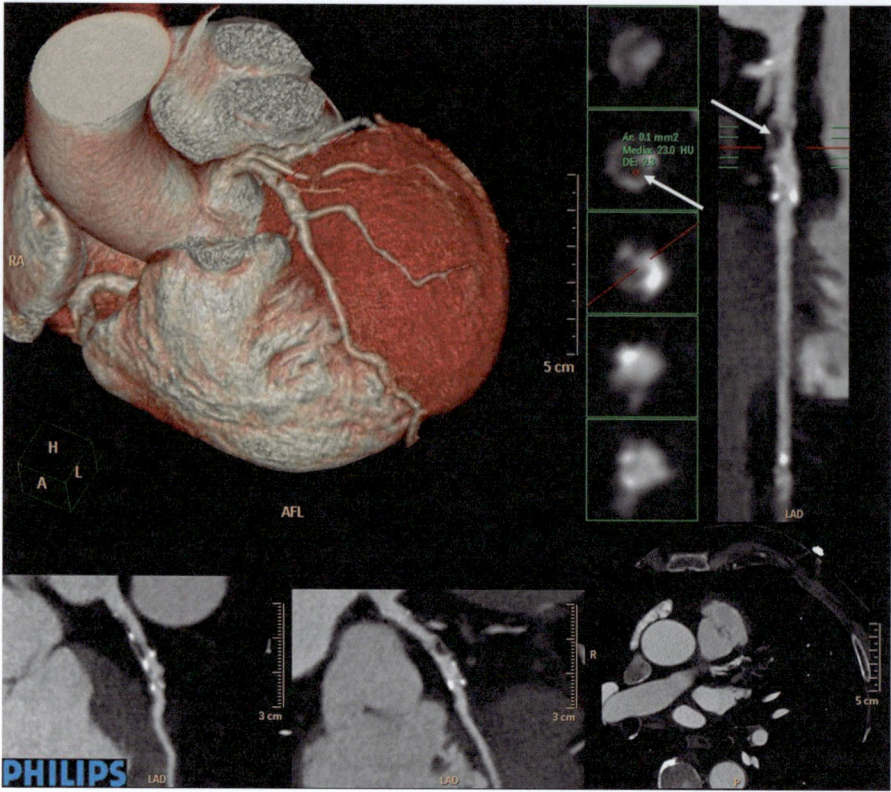

Fig. 10.24 Very low density signal of a coronary plaque (*arrows*), suggesting the presence of a necrotic core

plaque, which may indicate the presence of a necrotic core (see Fig. 10.24), which also occurs in vulnerable plaques.

Currently, most of the cardiac MDCT analysis devices have tools that permit the performance of the so-called virtual histology, which consists of an automatisation of the previously described process of HU quantification. These programmes perform an automatic detection of the borders of the plaque (both the inner luminal border and the external pericoronary border) (see Fig. 10.20) and assign a range of Hounsfield values to each tissue component, which are represented by shades of colour superimposed on the image of the atheroma plaque (see Fig. 10.25). Such

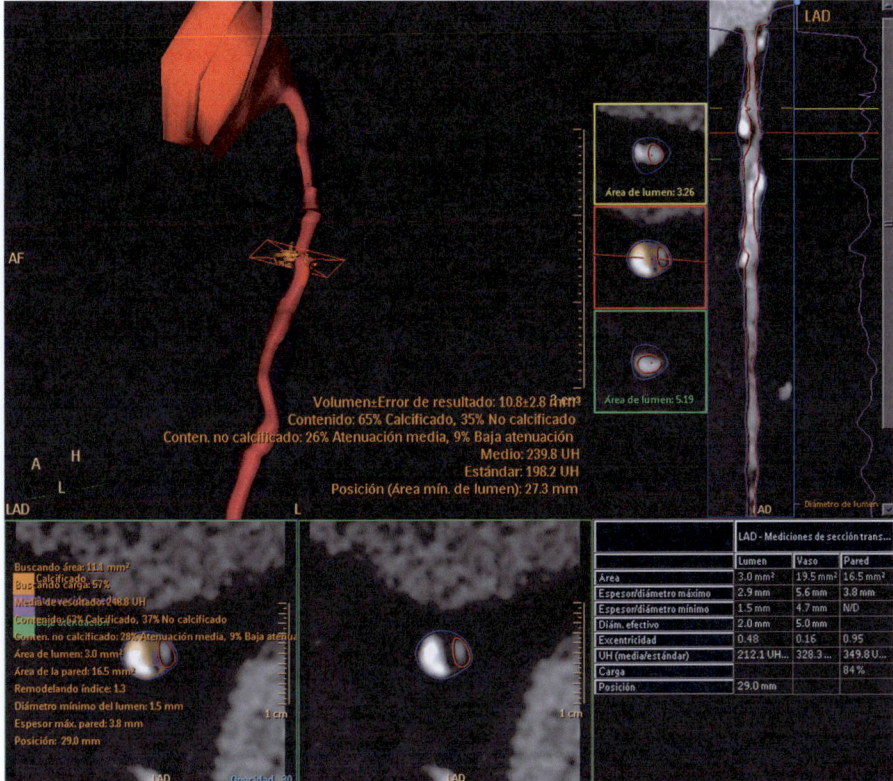

Fig. 10.25 Colour-coded analysis of signal intensities of coronary plaque components

systems allow not only the evaluation of the composition of the plaque but also the quantification of the volume of the plaque in an area affected by diffuse atherosclerosis.

Recommended Bibliography

1. Arbab-Zadeh A, Hoe J (2011) Quantification of coronary arterial stenoses by multidetector CT angiography in comparison with conventional angiography methods, caveats, and implications. JACC Cardiovasc Imaging 4:191–202
2. Leipsic J, Abbara S, Achenbach S, Cury R, Earls JP, Mancini GJ et al (2014) SCCT guidelines for the interpretation and reporting of coronary CT angiography: a report of the Society of Cardiovascular Computed Tomography Guidelines Committee. J Cardiovasc Comput Tomogr 8:342–358
3. Raff GL, Abidov A, Achenbach S, Berman DS, Boxt LM, Budoff MJ et al (2009) SCCT guidelines for the interpretation and reporting of coronary computed tomographic angiography. J Cardiovasc Comput Tomogr 3:122–136
4. Rinehart S, Vázquez G, Qian Z, Murrieta L, Christian K, Voros S (2011) Quantitative measurements of coronary arterial stenosis, plaque geometry, and composition are highly reproducible with a standardized coronary arterial computed tomographic approach in high-quality CT datasets. J Cardiovasc Comput Tomogr 5:35–43

MIX
Papier aus verantwortungsvollen Quellen
Paper from responsible sources
FSC® C105338

If you have any concerns about our products,
you can contact us on
ProductSafety@springernature.com

In case Publisher is established outside the EU,
the EU authorized representative is:
**Springer Nature Customer Service Center GmbH
Europaplatz 3, 69115 Heidelberg, Germany**

Printed by Libri Plureos GmbH
in Hamburg, Germany